AF323826

New Frontiers in Aging

New Frontiers in Aging

SPIRIT AND SCIENCE TO MAXIMIZE PEAK
EXPERIENCE IN YOUR 60S, 70S, AND BEYOND

Olga Brom Spencer, Ph.D.

With Medical Editing by Anna C. Freitag, M.D.
Foreword by Stacy Enyeart

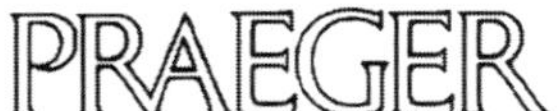

Westport, Connecticut
London

Library of Congress Cataloging-in-Publication Data

Spencer, Olga Brom.
    New frontiers in aging : spirit and science to maximize peak experience in your 60s, 70s,
    and beyond / Olga Brom Spencer.
        p. cm.
    Includes bibliographical references and index.
    ISBN 978–0–313–35933–0 (alk. paper)
1. Aging. 2. Longevity. I. Title.
RA776.75.S74 2008
613.2—dc22   2008029269

British Library Cataloguing in Publication Data is available.

Library of Congress Catalog Card Number: 2008029269
ISBN: 978–0–313–35933–0

First published in 2008

Praeger Publishers, 88 Post Road West, Westport, CT 06881
An imprint of Greenwood Publishing Group, Inc.
www.praeger.com

Printed in the United States of America

The paper used in this book complies with the
Permanent Paper Standard issued by the National
Information Standards Organization (Z39.48–1984).

10 9 8 7 6 5 4 3 2 1

The opinions and ideas of the authors expressed in this literary work are intended to provide
helpful and informative material on the subjects addressed in this publication. The authors
and publishers are not providing medical, legal, health-related, or any other kind of professional services in this book. The readers should consult with their medical, legal, health or
other competent professionals before adopting any of the ideas described in this book or
deducting inferences from it.

This book is highlighting the uniqueness of each individual, and, therefore, its contents cannot be interpreted as a panacea for any individual problems of aging or otherwise.

The authors as well as the publisher disclaim responsibility for any liability, losses, or other
damaging consequences that would result from a direct or indirect application of any of the
contents of this publication.

This book is dedicated to the memory of my parents whose wisdom and spirit of caring far survived the limitations of their physical presence.

Contents

Foreword

My credentials for writing the foreword to *New Frontiers in Aging* are not in gerontological psychology or associated disciplines, but rather are grounded in lifelong personal experience and practice of self-actualization, which this remarkable book serves to highlight: mainly, to live a life of purpose, success, vigor, and new possibilities that are not diminished by chronological age, change in life circumstances, or unavoidable losses.

To expect that this volume is a guide or a do-it-yourself manual for successful aging would be missing the author's point. A guide is something one has to follow to achieve a desired effect. The intention here is to provide information that inspires readers to increase awareness of their potentials and to design their own visions of aging in line with their individual uniquenesses.

The title itself, *New Frontiers in Aging*, expresses the author's thinking about the senior years: It is not a road of decline—even though existing illness and other conditions must be addressed and treated—but is rather a process of ongoing development. Although the nature of living entails more or less work in all ages, the author's concept of mobilizing the energy is not seen as an additional burden, but rather as a spontaneous process of self-development.

The concept of developing the self is not new; it was introduced and successfully applied to varied disciplines in the past. Spencer is reinventing this idea and proposing it as an age-appropriate way for quality living in senior years. Her invitation to a more creative life may lead to invigorating experiences that eventually climax in the achievement of greater self-awareness and humaneness. Such mind and spirit-elevating moments help validate the qualities that seniors possess, but were not encouraged or inspired to access during their busy days of middle age. Grandma Moses was a typical example of a self-actualizing woman. A farmer's wife for most of her life, she had time to realize only in later years what was her true vocation: painting.

It seems pertinent to say that the core of what Spencer is writing about is stemming from her own experiences. As an octogenarian and a survivor of many cancer surgeries and personal losses, she is pursuing a life of purpose, vigor, and ongoing personal development. It is true of all of us that once we connect, and are aware of our own deep nature, we are also able to understand simultaneously human nature, hopes, and concern of people in general.

For those readers who are already living a life of purpose and peak experiences, this book will validate that they are on the right track. For those who are on the way to self-actualization, the reading will provide much needed encouragement in their search for a purpose in later years. Life's fulfillment does not depend on the chronological age, but rather on the decisions of how we use time, energy, and talents and if we have a personal vision of our future. The author asks whether we are ready to grasp the opportunities for continuous growth or fail and grow old. The choices that we make influence our destinies.

It is encouraging to note the increase of energized seniors in our society: With *New Frontiers in Aging* and other evidence of this trend, a new perception and acceptance of advanced age is transforming a current mind-set about the senior population and creates new possibilities in the evolving universe of modern aging.

Stacy Enyeart
Executive Producer, Cable TV program *Ageless*
President, AARP Chapter, Westport/Weston, Connecticut
Recipient, AARP Community Service Award, Washington, D.C., 2005
Author, *America's World War II Home Front Heroes*
Co-Publisher, *Profiles Magazine*
Board Member, Connecticut Press Club
Board Member, National League of American Pen Women

Preface

Dum spiro-spero
As long as we breathe—we hope

—Latin Proverb

This book is about new frontiers in aging.

During the past decades, groundbreaking research in neuroscience, medicine, gerontological psychology, molecular biology, and particle physics transformed the perception of aging, as a process of decline and entropy, to an experience of new opportunities, renewal, and self-actualization. The possibility of extended youth and vigor, far beyond the sixth decade, is no longer a fantasy, but rather a new reality experienced by increasing numbers of seniors who are succeeding in postretirement careers and personal pursuits of happiness. They are the living proof that vitality and youth can be regenerated, as many aspects of growing old are under personal control. The profound truth is that our choices determine our destinies, and what happens to us during our lifetimes and after death depends on the choices that we make today.

This book provides inspiration and alternatives for a new experience of aging. Without alternatives we cannot make informed choices. Knowledge empowers us to select models of aging that are compatible with our personalities, talents, and abilities to adapt to changing life circumstances. There are countless differences in growing old because no two individuals are biologically identical.

Whatever lifestyle we choose for later years, it is important not only to experience successful aging physiologically, but also to derive meaning from an extended life span and use the newly acquired vigor and youth for purposes that will enhance our self-esteem and usefulness.

In searching for a new way of aging, we have to liberate ourselves from the power of obsolete beliefs that physiologic decline is inevitable and irreversible. These myths, deeply rooted in our minds by society, represent a barrier to the perception that regardless of chronological age, we have the competence of setting and reaching new goals in the process of living a purposeful life rather than leading an existence of mindless habit.

This book is an invitation to a journey opening new vistas for living that are inspired by spirituality and sciences. The only hero on this journey will be you, for it takes intellectual courage to be open to new opportunities and changes. The unexpected realities will inspire us to explore the road less traveled and look with anticipation to new horizons of life that can be truly magnificent.

Where does the journey begin?

The first step starts with our choice at the crossroad of Aging or Becoming.

Olga B. Spencer, Ph.D.

Acknowledgments

From the moment of its inception to the last page of the manuscript, this book was influenced by the comments of several colleagues, friends, and family members who, in spite of their busy schedules, put aside time for reading and reacting to the evolving chapters.

First and foremost, I would like to acknowledge the inspired contribution of Anna C. Freitag, M.D., leading endocrinologist, who authored an important chapter on prevention of diseases—"Impact of Lifestyles on Health"—that is a must-read chapter for seniors. I am also most grateful for her review of the accuracy of medical information in my chapters. Dr. Joel Singer, M.D., plastic surgeon of over 30 years, authored a chapter on "Modern Medicine and Rejuvenation," and his expert contribution is greatly appreciated. Also, I was impressed by the width and depth of knowledge of Nancy Ryan, M.S., R.D., C.D.E., whose chapter on nutrition—"Living Longer, Living Stronger" is an important enrichment to this book; it deserves credit for its thoroughness and wealth of information.

I greatly appreciated the assistance of Senior Editor of Praeger Press, of Greenwood Publishing Group, Debbie Carvalko, whose expert direction and help in all matters were instrumental in the smooth procession of the publication. I should not omit the work of Brian Foster, assistant editor, who facilitated the initial processing of the manuscript.

I am gratefully acknowledging the comments and critiques of Dr. Joan LaMontagne, psychologist and author, who made valuable recommendations to the manuscript. Special thanks are due to a longtime friend

Rhoda Gilinsky, former writer for the *New York Times,* whose professionalism stimulated my thinking to new heights of conceptual vision.

At last, but not least, I owe special thanks to my daughter Isabelle Breen, L.C.S.W., psychotherapist, who was the first reader of the manuscript and made invaluable suggestions to the sharpening of the book's focus. The expertise of an electronic engineer—my son C. J. Brom—stimulated my thinking in the field of higher energy.

The typing and the editing of the manuscript were tedious work. I would have been unable to have finished the manuscript in a timely fashion without the help of an outstanding Fairfield University student, Alexandra Gross, who braved the deadlines and delivered the chapters when needed.

And, of course, I am indebted to those seniors who preordered this book a long time before it was a finished product.

They all have my thanks for their faith in a new vision of aging.

1 ▪ ▪ ▪

The Fountain of Youth

Aging kills 100,000 people a day. There is a moral obligation to combat cancer, diabetes and other diseases. Aging is just the same.[1]

—Aubrey de Grey

From the earliest times, humankind has dreamed of the elixir of youth, the alchemistic potion that would extend human life and endow it with eternal youth. This dream is now becoming a reality, except in a dream, the wish magically comes true. In reality, the reversal of one's age and pursuit of timelessness require more than dreaming. It takes knowledge and action.

With the progress of research in molecular biology, medicine, psychology, and particle physics, the search for the fountain of youth brought forth many questions:

Can aging be delayed or avoided?
How far can we extend the human life span?
Can we preserve youth and vigor?

One of the initial hurdles on the way to conquer old age was the fact that no one could define the word old. Researchers found that aging, as a characteristic of chronological age, was misleading. Many older individuals were youthful, energetic, and productive, while others of the same chronological age were older psychologically and physiologically. It was necessary to look for other characteristics that would reliably define, measure, and establish a universal definition of old age.

Scientists put themselves to work and in the second half of the twentieth century announced the discovery of a new tool for measuring human age: the biomarkers. It is no longer chronological aging that counts, but biological indicators of physiological functioning that determine how old we are. They are assessing a person's cardiovascular capacity, short- and long-term memory, maximum breathing capacity, nerve conductive velocity, and performance of other organs. Currently, aging is no longer defined in general terms, but rather by the performance and health of particular organs. While some organs are aging, others may become gradually younger than their chronological age. For example, cells in the human body regenerate, but the change does not affect all organs equally. Skin replaces itself every month, liver tissue every six weeks, the stomach lining every five days, while the skeleton only once in three months. Thousands of new neurons are created daily from stem cells in the brain and spinal cord, reports Dr. Daniel Goleman in his groundbreaking book *Social Intelligence.*[2] Other cells, such as the heart cells, do not have the capacity to renew.

If the liver is polluted by toxins, its function regresses to older levels, but it can regenerate by detoxification and proper diet and become younger. In the human body, 98 percent of the atoms are renewed annually. Constant renewal keeps aging plastic and modifiable. It is our responsibility to preserve youth and vigor until the last possible moment when the rectangular survival curve declines toward the physiological end.

Plasticity is a word to remember. It is an umbrella for the physical, mental, and social markers of aging. It means that in a healthy person the lifespan or the functioning of organs in the body is not predetermined, inflexible, or fixed, but can be modified by the lifestyle we choose.

It is often erroneously believed that old age is a cause of chronic illness, such as emphysema, edema, congestive heart disease, neuropathy, diabetes, osteoarthritis, arteriosclerosis, or visual problems. In most cases, these conditions are self-induced and can be controlled or eliminated by personal determination, discipline, and perseverance, under medical supervision. It cannot be stressed enough that plasticity and lifestyle are in constant confrontation. Every action we take today is either increasing or decreasing our health and plasticity tomorrow.

The Roman philosopher Seneca conveyed that man does not die, he kills himself.[3] Poor diet, overeating, smoking, excessive use of alcohol, physical inactivity, overuse of drugs, and stress promote deterioration of the human organism.

This 2,000-year-old statement confronts us with tough choices. Do we prefer to pollute our bodies with cigarette smoke, an unhealthy diet, drugs, a sedentary lifestyle that reduces oxygen intake, or are we ready to value ourselves and protect our bodies so that they may thrive the way they were intended to, not only today but tomorrow and beyond?

Dr. Bernie S. Siegel, in his bestseller *Love, Medicine and Miracles,* highlights the healing power of love. He states, "The extent to which we love ourselves determines whether we eat right, get enough sleep, wear seatbelts, smoke, exercise, and so on. Each of these choices is a statement of how much we care about living. These decisions control about 90 percent of the factors that determine our state of health."[4]

When one of his patients was diagnosed with cancer, she asked whether he will tell her to stop smoking.

"No, I am going to tell you to love yourself. Then you will stop,"[5] said Siegel.

If we do not value and care for ourselves, who will? Love is an emotion that dissipates if it is not supported by an action; it means nothing if we do not transform it into practice. Protecting ourselves and our futures from unhealthy habits is a proof that regardless of our age, we count, we believe in ourselves, and we take our lives seriously enough to make a conscious effort not to waste them. Knowledge and the intention to do something are not enough. We have to take action to succeed.

Based on the pioneering work of a noted psychiatrist, Dr. Karen Horney, we all have a central inner force, common to all human beings, and yet unique to each of us, which, given a chance, is a deep source of growth. This core, the real self, is also our reserve of energy, love, and new potential.[6] This source had already been acknowledged 3,000 years ago by King David who referred to it as the "health of my countenance."[7]

Most people are not aware of the real self. We live life oriented toward external goals and do not have time to listen to the inner voice within us that leads us toward our true humaneness. Why have we lost connection to that core? Society rewards achievements that are often won at the cost of suppressing the real self. We are conditioned to look for rewards outside of us rather than to seek them inside ourselves.

In our busy lives pursuing external goals, from working to managing a daily routine, keeping in touch with the family and friends, volunteering, and so forth, we need to come to our inner selves to focus on what is going on and where we are spiritually. If we do not have that center, that sense of self, we are in trouble. We need to know where we are walking, what is up there ahead of us. "Follow your bliss," states influential mythologist Joseph Campbell. "There is something inside you that knows when you are in the center, that you are on the beam."[8]

We need to be aware of what we are doing to live consciously. Centering on the real self starts with answering questions: What counts at this stage of my life? What can I improve? What do I need, and what can I give?

One of the major steps forward is to give up blaming others for our circumstances and take responsibility for our lives. If we are not in charge of our aging, we are abdicating power over our precious independence to someone else who will control it. The statement "I am old" is a very common excuse for not living. We create a new experience of aging by the power of our thoughts that create a new image of our body and future.

Another step to conscious living is to seek private truth within ourselves. Horney reminds us to discern the real self from the pseudo-self, something that we pretend to be, but are not. People who are locked in the pseudo-self do not feel what they do: They smile to cover up sadness, they pretend to love when they have opposite emotions, or they are hiding behind a façade of self-sufficiency when they are yearning for attention and love. Some seniors, plagued by grief and loneliness following a loss, may be driven to empty pursuits of superficial value, that once attained, leave them dissatisfied and unfulfilled.

The question some seniors ask is how to reach the state of greater self-awareness. Where do they start? Some find the answer in daily prayer, mediation, inspirational reading, listening to quality music, or in creative imagery. The latter technique is increasingly popular because it can be practiced anywhere, anytime, provided one can find a quiet place to relax while sitting, reclining, or lying on one's back.

As a first step, settle into a comfortable position—close your eyes and focus on the genuine core in you, one that is timeless because it connects you to the eternal energy of the universe, penetrating everything within and outside of you. Think of something calm and healing. With every exhale, let the worries and stress leave your body. Imagine yourself resting in the warm sand on the shore and staring into the clear skies above you. You sense the universe expanding above you into the limitless, infinite space, and you are feeling enveloped by its protective peace and serenity. You may close your eyes or keep them open, whichever you prefer. Imagine yourself as a weightless being, floating in the warm breeze toward the blue skies above you, and as you are breathing, you inhale the creative energy of the universe. You are aware that you were born for a purpose, and that purpose is the fulfillment of your unique gifts. You feel the waves of energy filling your core, and you receive that energy as the universe's gift to you. You inhale the beneficial waves of energy and feel regenerated by them. As you are descending toward the peaceful beach, you feel generous, rested, and ready to pursue your uniqueness in whatever way you will decide. You are connecting with the real self as you are walking on the road toward the recognition of your spiritual identity.

The soul opens up if we pay attention to it. However, if you have difficulty imagining, a tape of guided imagery or meditation of your choice may be helpful. The connection to the real self is sometimes difficult because of emotional pollution in the mind, bad habits, disappointing experiences, pain, and stress that have corroded the access to the core of our inner selves. We need to regenerate and validate the essence of who we are: The truth is that connecting with the real self will bring us closer to wholeness and health.

Before we start the day in the morning and give into the routine of bad habits that pollute our lives, let us reconnect with the real self and become conscious of our loving potential. It is possibly the most important exercise we can do to elevate us above aging and entropy.

To care for ourselves is not a narcissistic endeavor, but rather a process of self-actualization and development of gifts and talents that were bestowed on us by nature. There is not a single person in the world who is not gifted, but there are many who resist to recognize their inherent potential and develop it.

Every time we care for ourselves and say "no" to pollutants, we are making a step in the right direction. Walking the road less traveled leads to rewards called independence, fulfillment, timelessness, and peak experiences.

■ ■ ■

One of the most essential conditions in aging is the physical plasticity. Without the ability to walk for health and care for ourselves, our independence would be seriously compromised. Fortunately, even very old seniors can sustain or improve their walking capacities.

Exciting data from *Runner's World* indicates that chronological age is not a reliable indicator of performance in marathon running. Increasing numbers of seniors have developed an interest in running in later years of life. One of them, 80-year-young Helen Klein, put her knitting needles down at the age of 55 and since then has finished 59 marathons and 132 ultramarathons. In 2003, she shattered the world marathon record for her age group. In Oregon, John Beeson, 90 years of age, set a new American record for 90-plus runners.[9] A memorable record held since 1908 was defeated not many years ago by a 65-year-old runner. The decisive predictor of physical performance is not age but practice.

If your doctor does not object to your walking, the benefits of practice accrue and health benefits increase. Loss of weight, lower blood pressure, increases in vital capacity, decreased cholesterol, and improvement of cardiac reserve are some of the health benefits of physical activity. The plasticity of the physical condition improves for all ages.

"Exercise is the closest thing to an anti-aging pill now available. It acts like a miracle drug and is free for the doing," says Robert N. Butler, M.D., president of the International Longevity Center—USA.[10] Even the old and weak have the capacity to increase their muscle mass, strength, balance, and walking ability, if they exercise regularly.

Butler recommends a simple, anti-frailty exercise that can be practiced at home.

1. Sit on a hard chair.
2. Cross your arms in front of your chest.
3. Get up without leaning forward.
4. Sit and repeat the exercise.

If you can do this exercise five times in 17 seconds, you are not frail.[11] If you do not succeed in achieving five sit-ups, do as many as possible. Practice every day and you will gradually increase and improve your physical fitness.

Physical frailty is one of the major reasons why men and women enter nursing homes. Frailty is an impairment of the physical abilities necessary for independent living that afflicts more than 3 million people in the United States.

While medical care is important for the prevention of frailty and disability, physical fitness is recommended by the National Institute on Aging as an essential factor in maintaining independence.[12]

Although doctors alert us to the consequences of inactivity, such as loss of muscle and balance, improper breathing, diabetes, and other ailments, 49 million people in the United States are sedentary, not engaging in physical activities.[13]

If you do not participate in any form of physical exercise, your answers to the following questions will help you to focus and decide on what is in your best interest.

Please check one:

1. I do not care if I become frail; aging cannot be stopped.
2. I made a resolution to walk every day, but for one reason or another I cannot keep it.
3. My neighborhood is not appropriate for walking.
4. I would like to walk, but I never seem to have enough energy.
5. I know that walking is good for my health, but after doing my other chores in the house and garden, I feel too tired.
6. I do not like to walk. Is there another exercise that would benefit my health?

If you answered number 1, you might be experiencing a depressive episode. You should consult your physician. If you are not depressed, but expect to get frail, your expectation will become your reality. Our beliefs hold great power over our bodies, and aging happens in our minds first.

If you answered number 2 or 3, it might be helpful to start with smaller steps rather than with a big goal. You can try walking on a treadmill, installed in a pleasant area of your home. Many people like to walk while watching TV or listening to music.

If you answered number 4, remember that physical activity increases energy, and sedentary life decreases it. Dr. S. Jay Olshansky, a longevity researcher from the University of Chicago, says that physical activity cuts the risk of dying by half.[14]

If you answered number 5, you do not need to walk. Dr. M.F. Roizen states that a 30-minute walk is equivalent to 30 minutes of gardening,

15 minutes of swimming, 20 minutes of tennis, and 17 minutes of hiking.[15] Dr. Gary Small suggests that rhythmic tasks such as sweeping, raking, mopping, and other household activities can burn calories if they are done routinely.[16]

If you answered number 6 and do not like walking, pedaling a bike now will be better than pedaling in a wheel chair later.

Are there limits to physical plasticity?

Physically active seniors can sustain the same performance for a very long time. However, there is a gradient and every year we can expect our physical performance to show some decrease. If maintaining performance takes ever more time and effort and exhausts our reserves, then we can choose to invest energy into physical activity in other areas. It is typical for successful aging that some activities decline while others increase. Yoga, tai chi, hydro exercise, and gentle resistance exercises are some of the activities that can be extended into the ninth decade.

■ ■ ■

Until very recently it was assumed that intelligence declined with advanced age. This belief was proven to be wrong by many experiments in which it was demonstrated that intelligence is plastic and its decline is avoidable. Moreover, in addition to the mental activity of the brain, every cell and molecule have intelligence. Our thoughts are followed by a chemical reaction that carries information from the brain into every part of the body. The mind-body connection is a groundbreaking process that allows us to influence our health by the way we think.

One of the well-known experiments by a group of researchers, J. K. Plemon, S. I. Willis, and P. B. Baltes, proved that even seniors in their 80s can improve mental functioning. Exposure to intellectual training resulted in marked improvements in fluid intelligence in the experimental group, while seniors in the control group did not improve.[17]

Maintaining a mental functioning in good shape requires the continued use of the mind, engagement in cognitive activities. The danger of retirement or inactive life cannot be underestimated. For many people, employment was a major source of social and mental stimulation, and they have to look for new types of brain exercise. The old proverb ''use it or lose it'' proves to be true. Pablo Picasso, who remarried in his 70s and started a new career in ceramics, was known for saying, ''It takes a long time to become young.''[18]

Variation in intelligence is noticeable even among seniors who are our relatives, colleagues, neighbors, and friends. Why are some of them showing intellectual decline, while others' minds are as sharp as they have always been?

People are creatures of habit. Familiar tasks may lead to repetitions and, consequently, to mental laziness. In order to simplify thinking, some seniors tend to put incoming information into categories to better organize and control them. Once categorized, they become gradually obsolete. To remain mentally fit, we need to respond to new stimuli in a fresh way to avoid repetitious reactions and stimulate the brain with ever new responses.

Increasing numbers of research findings indicate that mentally active people, who are involved with life, are growing new dendrites, those tree-like filaments that are facilitating communication between the brain cells. It appears that dying neurons can be reinforced by new small neurons that are encouraging the brain mechanism to be active in old age. To sustain a mental functioning involves a life commitment to oneself, not only once in a while but as a matter of daily activity. It does not matter whether you do crossword puzzles, learn a new language, or go back to college. Just do it!

■ ■ ■

Plasticity of memory is another area that was believed to decline with advancing age and was thought to be irreversible. The truth is that there is great variability among seniors of the same chronological age, depending on their cognitive activities and health.

There are different types of memory: Episodic memory, which relates to events from childhood, is very stable. Procedural memory, such as driving a car, is not affected much by time. Semantic memory, remembering language, survives aging quite well. The most frequent complaints refer to short-term memory and access to stored information. However, improvement of short-term memory was demonstrated by Harvard psychologist Dr. Ellen J. Langer in a well-documented experiment with 80-year-old residents of a nursing home: They were divided into two groups and instructed to memorize recent events. One group was rewarded for remembering; the other was not. Memory improved in the group of seniors that was rewarded. The difference between the two groups was striking. The study indicated that short-term memory is plastic, and it is possible to reverse its loss. Seniors can improve their memory if they overcome mental laziness, are mindful of their thoughts, and use their cognitive capacity daily.[19]

Complaints of poor memory may accompany functional depression, and they disappear when depression is treated. Loss of memory may be a sign of more serious disorders, such as dementia or Alzheimer's disease; it is vital not to postpone a visit to a physician when forgetfulness is interfering with daily living.

▥ ▥ ▥

Another serious problem affecting seniors is social disengagement. It is a process of gradual withdrawal from interaction with people and environment, either because some seniors live alone and have no family members to visit them or, in some circumstances, aging people do not have enough energy for what it takes to interact.

Social isolation tends to increase with advanced age and results in the decline of functioning and energy and an increase in entropy and death in an institutionalized setting. Health problems are frequently reported in seniors who live alone and do not have any contact with family or friends. To live is not the same as being alive. In order to stay alive, we need to be actively involved in life.

In a series of experiments, Langer demonstrated that considerable social and health benefits result from interaction with other people. She tested two groups of 80-year-old seniors in a nursing home. The members of one group were told to relax, watch TV, and ask the staff whenever they needed something. The other group's members were told to live as if they were at home, to interact with others, and to be responsible for watering plants in the residence. After 19 months, the control group was found to be much happier, active, and self-initiating; the death rate was 15 percent. In the leisure group, 30 percent of the seniors died, and the remainder showed marked signs of helplessness.[20] If seniors cannot participate in making decisions, they learn to be helpless and lose autonomy as well as a reason to live. The ability to make one's own choices is essential for well-being at any age. Seniors who can control their lives age much better than those who have abdicated control to others. The old saying "to rest is to rust" is true not only for the body but also for the mind and social skills.

Daniel Goleman, who revolutionized the definition of human connections in his book *Emotional Intelligence,* discusses evidence that positive interaction can boost the immune system.[21] Thanks to neuroscience, experts were able to observe brain activity during the process of feeling. One person's inner state affects the other person's emotional receptors. We are forming brain-to-brain bridges all the time. Goleman is advising us to avoid so-called "toxic" relationships that may have harmful consequences for us because stress and anxiety produce cortisol in our bodies that suppress the immune system. On the other hand, positive interaction reinforces the immune system in a great way.[22]

Nobody is an island. We are all interconnected. Two persons can communicate from within, without words, radiating outward positive emotions that will lead to mutuality and unification. We cannot communicate unless we are willing to share ourselves. There must be intention to share. Everybody has the capacity to communicate, if we overcome resistance and connect with the inner self.

▓ ▓ ▓

Preserving plasticity of physical dexterity, intelligence, memory, and cognitive performance is a matter of choice. It does not depend on one's age, but on practice and lifelong commitment to oneself every day if we want to keep our vigor and youth. As soon as we begin to pay attention to any function in our bodies, a transformation takes place. If we withdraw awareness from the body, we are regressing from the spiritual to mechanical level that is gravitating to entropy. As our chronological ages increase, so does our wisdom, creativity, capacity for love and compassion, and other talents that we did not have time to develop during our years of employment and child rearing. While practicing plasticity, let us revive the connection to the heart by loving what we are doing as we are *becoming* more aware, fulfilled, and completed.

Remember that we and our real selves are partners. We have to communicate, negotiate, compromise, but we can never abdicate what is the best part of us.

And what happens if we do not cooperate and stand for ourselves? The answer can be found in T.S. Eliot's profound statement: "If we haven't the strength to impose our terms on life, we must accept the terms that life offers to us."[23]

To walk the path of a new experience of aging is a matter of choice.

2 ▪ ▪ ▪

The Fourth Age

Two old friends meet after a long separation.
"You look great" one says. "How old are you?"
The other answers, "How old would I be if I didn't know my age?"

—Popular anecdote

If someone asks "how old are you?" which of the three ages of man comes to your mind? The chronological, biological, or psychological?

As is well known, *chronological age* is the official age that cannot be changed. However, how old we really are is influenced by the biological and psychological ages determining where we stand among our contemporaries, as well as how we define ourselves as individuals. To state chronological age is often misleading because age characteristics of only very few individuals are evenly represented on the average statistical tables; according to such researchers as Caleb E. Finch, James F. Fries, and Laurence M. Crapo, scores of most seniors are scattered around the average, reflecting the variation from the norm, as well as the growing diversity of the aging population.[1]

The *biological age,* also called the age of our arteries, is influenced by lifestyles that either improve or undermine health and increase or decrease proximity to death. Plasticity and performance of individual organs show how young we really are. Those biofactors are not fixed, but can be improved by diet, exercise, and other means. Michelangelo is often used as an example of young biological age. He was the architect of St. Peter's Basilica in Rome from age 72 until his death at the age of 88. Galileo Galilei, who published his masterpiece *Dialogues Concerning Two New Sciences* at the age of 74, is another example. Noah Webster completed his famous *Dictionary of the English Language* at the age of 70, and Konrad Adenauer took over defeated Germany at the age of 73 and built it into an economic power up to his 85th year. They all were biologically young men.

Psychological age is the major factor in our adaptive capacities, how well we can adjust to new life circumstances. Two hundred years ago, Charles R. Darwin discovered that survival of the species did not depend on their intelligence or strength, but rather on their successful adaptation to changing environments.

Adaptability to a changing world is a great personal asset at any age, but it is especially important for seniors. They spend enormous amounts of mental, physical, and psychological energy dealing with changes due to losses. Whether it is the loss of a spouse, friend, income, beloved pet, home, or a limb due to disability, adaptation to change requires ongoing readiness to deal with new life circumstances.

More often than not, our three ages are not well coordinated and are on different age levels. A 60-year-old Clark Gable and many other movie stars played 20-year younger lovers. Cary Grant became a father for the first time at the age of 60. Charlie Chaplin fathered his last child at the age of 72. Marlene Dietrich seduced the public as a 62-year-old grandmother with the appearance of a 40-year-old woman. Picasso remarried at the age of 79 and stayed in the relationship until his death at 91. There are millions of less well-known seniors, whose chronological age is more advanced than their youthful appearances, revealing a creative, productive, and fulfilled individual. On the other hand, there are millions of seniors who appear much older and carry the burden of accumulating years with obvious pain and difficulties. Time is passing equally for the younger and older looking, but everybody metabolizes time and experiences differently. Some are using time for renewal, and some are giving into entropy.

My encounter with Colette, a French novelist in the early 1950s in Paris, was a striking evidence of the psychological imbalance of the three ages of mankind. When we met, she was a frail woman in a wheelchair. From her wrinkled face surrounded by frizzy gray hair shined a pair of young lively eyes. She asked about my age, and when I answered that I was 20 years old, she nodded. "When I was twenty, I felt very old. Now I am old and feel young." Her eyes sparkled like stars and her life-inspiring smile mirrored ageless inner youth. Even though she was disabled, she was involved in life with a contagious vigor.

To know one's *real* age, the way one feels, is important because aging begins in the mind. Every thought influences cells in the body, informing them whether they are young or old. This extraordinary communication system between mind and body can indeed influence one's organism either toward youth or decline. Colette was young because she believed that she was young, and her thoughts were changing her biology. The same dynamic applies to all of us: If we believe that we must age because it is unavoidable, our cellular systems will comply with such a message. To become young at any age starts with giving up myths that aging cannot be delayed.

People's three ages are accepted by the public as well as by the professional community more or less as the norm. Yet, there is another age that is more visible, convincing, and representative of how the world sees us. I call it our fourth age: the appearance.

We might not know what a person's breathing capacity, liver function, chronological age, or nerve conductive velocity is, but the appearance reveals into what real age category such a person belongs. When seniors are asked about their ages, and they state the truth, often the reaction is "you look much younger," or "I would never have guessed that you are that old."

The age of our appearance is important because it places us into a generational context where we belong biologically, psychologically, but not chronologically. A black cleaning woman who decided to attend college at the age of 60, and received her Bachelor of Arts degree at the age of 72, was displaced in the group of her church contemporaries who did not know quite how to relate to her. She was becoming younger, and they were aging. The educational process changed her appearance and demeanor from the inside out.

Recently, during a social gathering, I met a good-looking woman with her escort. To my dismay, she introduced him as her son. The bald, wrinkled, overweight man was the son of a woman who looked a decade younger than he did. She was an active realtor, always on the go, he was a computer operator who described himself as a "couch potato." This uneven couple demonstrated the statement of Dr. S. Jay Olshansky, longevity researcher at the University of Illinois in Chicago: "Exercise is the closest thing we have to a fountain of youth."[2] This and similar quotes are becoming the axiom of health-conscious people of all ages.

General studies, lasting several years, have shown that being active and exercising can counteract the loss of muscle, reduce blood pressure and inflammation, improve cholesterol levels, and energize the brain activities.

This discrepancy between chronological age and youthful appearance is accepted by the general public with some ambivalence. Why is it so? Creation of younger looks, absence of wrinkles, double chins, gray hair, and sagging body parts, which are all characteristics of old age, has not yet been accepted as part of a usual aging process. The values of our society promote authenticity and truth, and to correct what Mother Nature left to decay is against the principle of so-called "graceful aging" within the generational lines.

Yet, it is paradoxical that our society values youth and the dynamic contribution young people bring to the gross national product, culture, sports, technology, and other areas of society. With the increasing numbers of aging Americans and the decreasing numbers of young people who have to support them, it seems inevitable that seniors will have to work longer and keep their health and independence longer as well. Younger appearances are helping in successful adjustment in postretirement careers. Increasing numbers of aging executives, seen in the offices of plastic surgeons, are discretely resorting to procedures that will prolong their youthful appearances and minimize the signs of aging to a realistic minimum.

Our fourth age leads to a growing new industry of rejuvenation. Increasing numbers of busy plastic surgeons, makeover wizards, hair replacement specialists, dentists, cosmetic products, and skin care centers are evidence that the appearance is gradually becoming a significant part of seniors' lives. Each year, millions of Americans undergo surgical procedures to improve their appearances, and billions are spent on cosmetics to help people look younger.

A real couple, identified by the fictitious names Ben and Lea, was devastated by prostate and breast cancer, respectively, shortly after retirement. They were fortunate to survive, but confrontation with death left them both in a depressed mood. Then, they attended a conference by a well-known lecturer, Dr. Wayne W. Dyer, and this experience changed their perspectives on life; they decided to rebuild their future.

Before starting a new career at the age of 67, Lea underwent liposuction of a double chin, silicon filling of facial lines, and her gray hair was changed to the natural blonde she used to be. Her face revealed her new age of 50. Lea's psychological and cosmetic makeover inspired Ben to work on his appearance as well. He joined a fitness club, determined to shed a few excessive pounds and rebuild his flabby muscles. With rejuvenated appearances, they dedicated time to a national organization for the prevention of cancer. They were also active in fundraising for the same cause.

When a friend asked Lea about her noticeably younger appearance, she said, "You cannot pretend to be young. Imitation is a fake that nobody believes. You must become young at heart and adjust the appearance with the real age inside."

The Human Genome Project in the United States established that only 25 percent of aging is determined by our genes, and 75 percent results from our choices, behavior, and environmental factors. This empowers us to control our health and appearance to a much larger extent than it was thought possible in the past.[3]

Surveys of people who underwent medical "makeovers" show that the experience of external change can also rejuvenate the person's internal perception of self. Studies at Harvard Medical School, led by Dr. Itzhak Aharon, demonstrated that subjects responded positively to beautiful faces as manifested by the release of dopamine to the brain.[4]

However, not everybody is ready for a cosmetic procedure. Those who believe in a natural approach to rejuvenation might benefit from the following steps:

- Adequate sleep,
- Exercise,
- Healthy nutrition,
- Internal and external hydration,
- Minimal exposure to the sun, and
- Consultation with a dermatologist or plastic surgeon regarding nonsurgical or surgical procedures.

■ BEAUTY SLEEP

It is estimated that some 100 million Americans suffer from insomnia, causing irritability, fatigue, loss of productivity, and tired appearance.[5] To establish a better sleeping pattern in an otherwise healthy senior, the following steps are helpful:

- Take a brief walk or exercise two hours before dinner.
- Serve the last meal of the day no later than between 6 and 7 P.M.
- Consume a light dinner. Avoid coffee or beverages that interfere with sleep.
- Indulge in low-key activities one hour before retiring to bed, such as reading, nonviolent TV, meditation, personal care, listening to music, and so forth. Avoid stressful conversations or telephone calls.
- Your bed should be comfortable, the bedroom well ventilated, and the décor, lights, and sounds conducive to sleep.
- Sleep before midnight is more restorative. Turn off the lights and TV at 10 P.M., and say a prayer or give thanks for the past day.
- If you awake during the night, do not watch TV. Try self-hypnosis[6] to fall asleep again. If you do not succeed, consult a physician if a sleeping pill would temporarily help. Do NOT solve problems at night; do not worry. Do not force sleep; it would produce an opposite reaction. Some seniors find that reading or listening to relaxing tapes lulls them to sleep.
- If sleeplessness is the result of anxiety, anger, guilt, or other emotions, the resolution of such states should be initiated, preferably with professional help.
- Some professions do not allow the development of a regular sleep pattern. Actors, musicians, nurses, or late-night lovers would benefit from establishing their own individual sleeping habits that assure regular and sufficient amounts of rest.
- Sleep is essential because, during sleep, the consciousness is blanked out and the metabolism slows down to recharge the energy threshold.

■ EXERCISE

We already know that exercise is the fountain of youth. The MacArthur Foundation Study shows that ''happy activities'' promote successful aging. If an exercise is too strenuous, or we do not like it, we will not persevere in it. Here is a choice of activities, one of which you might like to practice on a regular basis:[7]

Walking	Racquet Sport	Gardening
Jogging	Dancing	Dog Walking
Swimming	Aerobics	Skiing
Cycling	Workout Equipment	Ice-Skating

A popular sport that has been resurrected is pool walking. This walking is done in a swimming pool for five to seven minutes and was found to strengthen muscles and improve circulation.

Whatever your choice, practice at least one sport or activity that you enjoy.

■ HYDRATION

Our bodies are made of about 62 percent water of total body weight. Dr. Phyllis A. Balch and Dr. James R. Balch recommend that we drink at least eight glasses of water per day.[8] Seniors are at constant risk of dehydration because they have significantly lower sensation for thirst. Prepare eight glasses of water or juices in the morning, and check whether they are empty in the evening.

Good appearance depends on proper hydration. Our connective tissues contain substances that keep our skin elastic and moisturized. We also need to hydrate skin on the face and body through the use of hydrating creams that are available in many brands in pharmacies and special stores.

■ NUTRITION

Many seniors eat poorly for a variety of reasons. Without proper nutrition or diet, one's health and appearance may decline. Because of the importance of what we eat, a special chapter is dedicated to this vital subject (see Chapter 7).

■ SUN EXPOSURE

Exposure to too much sun can lead to prematurely aged skin, cause cataracts, and suppress the immune function. Ultraviolet rays can lead to melanoma, a skin cancer that may become fatal if not detected in time. We should always apply a sunscreen and wear a large hat and sunglasses.

Consult your physician if you are on sun-adverse medication.

▓ CONSULTATION WITH PROFESSIONALS

Whether you consider a surgical or nonsurgical procedure, you should be an informed customer: Find a well-recommended, professional member of The American Board of Plastic Surgery or of American Society of Plastic and Reconstructive Surgeons. Before any procedure, ask questions about the cost, the intervention, and the results. Chapter 9 provides detailed information on rejuvenation procedures.

Consider the consequences of any procedure. The younger you look, the more will be expected of you. You might lose some of your old friends, but will attract younger people.

To get a bonus of an additional 10 or 20 years of life is a gift not to be wasted. With new opportunities come new duties. It is the responsibility of every human being to aspire to do something worthwhile to make this world a better place than the one he or she found.

We can hardly fulfill such a goal unless we know why to survive. What is your purpose in life?

3 ▪ ▪ ▪

The Purpose

> If I can stop one heart from breaking
> I shall not live in vain
> If I can ease one life the aching
> Or cool one pain
> Or help one fainting robin
> Unto his nest again
> I shall not live in vain.[1]

> —Emily Dickinson

Why Survive? Growing Old in America is a Pulitzer Prize–winning book by Robert N. Butler, M.D., founding director of the National Institute on Aging.[2]

AARP retired president Horace B. Deets seconded Butler. "The result of longevity is that seniors have a bonus of 30 years of life. The challenge is what to do with 30 years? More years for what purpose?"[3]

The population of the United States reached a new milestone, 300 million people in 2006. By the year 2030, almost 30 percent of Americans will be 65 years old or older. Are we ready for such a dramatic change in our demography?[4]

In a survey of seniors at an AARP chapter in Connecticut in 2000, only about one-third of seniors stated that they have plans for the future. Nearly 70 percent reported that they do not have plans, or have vague plans, want to enjoy themselves, rest, and have no obligations.[5]

Our society programmed us to follow a blueprint from the moment of birth to the day we retire. Rituals and normative expectations, such as birthday celebrations, sweet 16 parties, confirmations and Bar Mitzvahs, graduations from school, first employment, dating, getting married and raising children, retiring and dying, are directing us to pass smoothly through life without disturbing the general societal flow. These accepted perceptions of human life are challenged by new realities of aging in the twenty-first century. All of a sudden, following retirement, 20–30 years of unstructured life are awaiting us without any normative roles. Nobody tells us what to do or what is expected of us.

Social planners are searching for new models of aging for seniors, but no one paradigm suits the growing masses of aging people, some of whom are ready to work and live and others to grow old because they refuse to grow. Some sociologists refer to seniors as the pioneers of a new era, exploring the waste territory of possibilities for their development and establishment of new systems of exchange and productivity. On the other hand, many seniors feel they are persons without a role because society considers that only work, volunteering, and education are normative activities assumed to increase self-esteem.

What do seniors really want?

The truth is that they are searching for a lifestyle that would be very different from the experience of their parents. A baby boomer told me,

> When I awake in the morning, I want to know that the day has meaning. I could not live the way my mother did, settled in a daily routine, day after day. She used detachment to escape pains of aging and thoughts of death. She never experienced herself, not even for a moment. She died without being aware of what was happening.[6]

The definition of successful aging is in many ways the same as the definition of successful life. Aging well is a skill that requires awareness of self, development of a goal, and a strategy to reach that goal. Most researchers agree that life without purpose, conscious or unconscious, tends to lead to crises.

Religious historian Samuel Brandon states that "there can be no more urgent task than that of resolving the dilemma of the meaning... of man's life in time."[7]

Search for meaning is reflected by the history of humankind:

Throughout human cultures, legends inform us of heroes who undertook dangerous journeys to discover their purpose in life: Moses went to Mount Sinai to return with the Ten Commandments. Jesus Christ came with the message of universal love over hatred. In modern times, Florence Nightingale braved great obstacles to reform hospital care. On each of these fantastic missions, the heroes transcended themselves, and the experience transformed them from a normal mortal person into an immortal being. They gave part of themselves for a higher purpose that had a major impact on humanity.

We are not different from the ancient heroes. Each of us is a unique creature able to do innovative things that nobody else could conceive. Some of us are aware of our special talents and are using them, or hope to use them when life circumstances will allow it. Some others are wondering what their special gifts might be, or what they would like to do during the last two to three decades of their lives.

The opportunities for doing something new are endless. Joseph Campbell said "that everyone has a potential, and the mission in life is to live that potentiality."[8] How do we do it?

Search for any new potential starts with an inward journey on the way to discovery of the real self. It is what Plato meant when he said, in "Euthydemus," that "a man who would be happy must not only have good things but must also use them: There is no advantage to merely having them."[9]

Since the earliest of times, men and women have had an innate tendency to improve themselves, to improve their living conditions, to do something new, which moved humanity forward, step by step. The artists in the caves of Lascaux or Cro-Magnon were not paid for their amazing designs on the walls of the caverns. They did it because the inner forces of their talents empowered them to do something different beyond the daily struggle for survival.

A Nobel Prize–winning biologist, Albert Szent-Györgyi, concluded his research with a groundbreaking statement that there is a universal drive in all human organisms at the cellular level, as well as in the total organism, that has the tendency to improve itself. He gave a solid backing to the concept of organism actualizing function.[10]

Carl R. Rogers stated that human beings, like every other living organism, plant or animal, have an inherent tendency to develop all their capacities in ways that serve to maintain or enhance the organism. This is a reliable tendency, which, when free to operate, moves human beings toward what is termed growth, maturity, and life achievement. This process has been found to be true in the psychological realm also. Given a reasonable climate for growth, the tendency to further actualize the organism can be realized or can even overcome obstacles and pain.[11]

George T. Ainsworth-Land states in his book *Grow or Die* that the nature of a cell is *not* something that *is*, but something forever in the process of *becoming*. It is not wholly determined, but it plays a great part in determining itself.[12]

Influenced by biological evidence of universal improvement of mankind, noted psychologist Abraham H. Maslow developed a clinical approach that was helpful in orienting an individual toward the exploration of his or her real self. He stated that once we begin to search for inward development, facts often point in a direction; they are vectorial:

> Facts just don't lie there like pancakes, just doing nothing. They are, to a certain extent, signposts which tell us what to do. They call for, they have a demand character, and they even have a "requiredness." Self-actualization can now be defined quite operationally as intelligence... leading us to a full humanness.[13]

When our ancestors were just hominids chiseling stone tools, it was hardly possible to predict that one day their posterity would progress to the construction of spaceships that would carry them to the moon and beyond. This evolutionary development, during thousands of years, highlights the fact that each of those individuals had drives that could not be suppressed. Rather than rest, they followed the universal urge to do something new, to improve their conditions, to self-actualize.

When the fight for survival was no longer a dominant factor during the early days of the agricultural revolution, the creativity and the imagination of individuals could be manifested through such activities as arts and philosophy. The mysterious force of self-development motivated the early people to express themselves creatively, seeking to understand and fulfill their unique roles in life.

Are we different from our ancient predecessors?

Part of the answer may be found in research exploring human drive and self-actualization on the cellular and molecular levels, as well as by the development of the brain.

Neurology Nobel Laureate Sir John Eccles stated that the "power of the brain is endless." There is no dispute among rational experts that we use only about 10 percent of the brain's power. Sir Eccles thought that even this low number is too high and said, "How can we calculate a percentage of infinity?"[14] It is awesome to imagine what potential each of us carries and yet uses it so scarcely. The brain contains 10 billion neurons and 120 billion glial cells. What kind of miracle awaits mankind if we think of our future role in the universe?

Even though we use only a fraction of our brain power and potential, the richness of our creative resources is sometimes unexpectedly revealed to us under certain circumstances. For example, when we have to fight for our lives, experience a religious epiphany, or are overpowered by the emotion of great love, then a tremendous reserve of energy, stored in our cores, is spontaneously released, and we experience a peak moment of insight into our potency and power.

Postretirement years provide ideal conditions for the further development of our potentials: We have more time for introspection, wisdom for appreciation of further reaches of human nature, and a desire to pursue something meaningful, to discover or develop our dormant talents. In order to find something new, we have to leave behind the old beliefs that no longer work for us and go in quest of a germinal idea, which will have the potential to lead us to an activity that will give a new dimension to our lives. Because so much of our former programming was unconscious, we have to learn that the most powerful weapon against aging is our consciousness.[15]

There are some among us who have doubts about the purpose of life and its meaning as we are aging. Sometimes we lose courage to live or feel unable to love. We may dislike ourselves, or even think that our lives were wasted and that it is too late for a new beginning because we are too old. All those experiences are the result of our failures to address the humanness and potential in our real selves, which calls for reconnection, no matter on what small level, and no matter at what age.

It is never too late to start something new. Harry Bernstein, born in 1910, was devastated when his wife of 67 years died. "There was much emptiness, and I had to find something to fill in the gap. I was looking for a home," he said.[16]

He found his home when he started to write about his childhood. After he finished his memoirs, *The Invisible Wall,* he offered the manuscript to several publishers, but they all declined. Mr. Bernstein was 96 years of age when Random House accepted and published his book. It was an instant success. When the *New York Times* interviewed him in 2007, Mr. Bernstein said, "I had to live to 90 because I was not ready to write the book when I was younger."[17] He suggested that people have to live until an advanced age in order to realize "a potential that lurks in them."[18] To start a new way of life is not given for free.

■ ■ ■

What are the activities of American seniors in general? According to John W. Rowe and Robert L. Kahn, one-third of seniors work for pay until a very advanced age. We know that many lawyers, physicians, artists, actors, and writers never retire, but pursue their careers throughout life. One-third of seniors volunteer in churches, hospitals, schools, and in not-for-profit organizations. Others provide much needed services to their family members or friends. Such activities are meaningful and purposeful and increase self-esteem in those who volunteer. The authors indicate that "any activity, paid or unpaid, that generate goods or services of economic value is productive."[19] Volunteering is an important attribute enhancing successful adaptation to aging: It was evidenced by a meta-analysis of 36 studies covering 25 years of research. It pointed to the significant increase in well-being among volunteers. Studies have shown that those individuals who have a purpose outside of themselves, clear goals, and structure in their everyday lives have a chance of living longer, improved quality lives.[20]

However, some seniors have difficulties in adjusting to life after retirement or following the loss of a lifelong partner. They are searching for a new reason to live. It is quite common to experience emptiness until a new adjustment is reached. What sometimes appears as laziness or a lack of motivation may be in reality inner deadness caused by pain and suffering that existed inside the core for years. It may signal a depressive episode that is hindering further adjustment to a new life; consultation with a professional can clear the mind from concerns, whether a treatment is needed or not.

Depression was treatable already in antiquity. According to writings dating from A.D. 200, Greek physician Ephesios successfully treated depressed patients with natural waters from an alkaline spring, which contained lithium. Interestingly, when lithium was discovered in 1818, it revolutionized the treatment of affective disorders in the United States. Depression can be cured by a variety of means, including pharmacology and psychotherapy.

Dr. Bernie S. Siegel expressed, in his book, a different opinion regarding treatment.

> The fundamental problem most patients face is an inability to love themselves, having been unloved by others during some crucial part of their life. The ability to love one self, combined with the ability to love life, enables us to improve the quality of life. Unconditional love is the most powerful stimulant of the immune system. The truth is that love heals.[21]

It is never too late to reconnect with the live force of real self, that central inner core common to all human beings that is the source of love, healing, and growth.

Harry Bernstein did not waste his time; he started to write a new book, *The Dream*. He did not write it under any self-imposed pressure. He said that he indulges in the luxury of writing when he feels like it, just as when he is hungry, he sits down and eats a meal. He loves what he is doing.

To know why to live is vital in all ages, but it is even more important in later years. Who needs us? Who loves us and whom do we love? Where can we make a positive difference? For it is awareness of ourselves and of our purposes that keeps us fulfilled. To start a new way of life is not free. We have to want it, plan it, and acquire it with patience and effort.

What happens when some of us are not willing to make the effort that living requires?

If nothing counts, and there is nothing to hope for, we are sending a message to the cells in our bodies that they should give up also. Every thought, positive or negative, is transformed by one's organism into either a beneficial or destructive chemical reaction that influences the biochemistry of one's body. The positive thoughts boost the immune system and regenerate health and vigor. Negative thoughts undermine the immune system and precipitate depression and decline. Thoughts are mighty allies because they can change perception of the environment and experiences by the power of positive thinking. Amazing liberation can be achieved by a conscious decision to use one's inherent talents and skills for a good cause.

Sometimes we notice that we attract people or events that are instrumental in the realization of our causes. On the other hand, when we follow destructive impulses, obstacles often appear in the way, hindering progress to our unsuspected declines.

Mrs. X. was a promising author, mother, and wife that could have a wonderful life if she was not an alcoholic. Her attempts to extricate herself from dependency on liquor in varied treatment facilities temporarily helped, but she relapsed periodically into alcohol abuse after several weeks of sobriety. Her desperate family organized an intervention during which Mrs. X. consented to commit herself once more to a reputed clinic. But soon after the admission, she got frustrated by the rules and signed herself out. She stormed out of the residence by slamming the door because the administrator declined to provide transport to the train. On that cool, fall evening, she walked angrily to the rural station alone. As she was approaching the platform, the train arrived. She assumed that the conductor would wait for her, but he apparently did not see her and the train left for New York without her. It was the last train of the day. Nobody was there to help, no taxi or other passengers (it was before cell phones were invented). Mrs. X. sat on the bench, shivering in the cold breeze. "What am I doing here?" she asked herself. "Why am I not with my husband and children?" She suddenly realized that the last train was her last chance. As she started to walk to the treatment residence, she was no longer an angry woman, but a person who realized, for the first time in her life, that there is something, or somebody, more powerful than herself. When the door of the residence opened, she asked humbly: "May I be readmitted?"

Mrs. X. not only completed the program, but she returned home to her family, started to write again, and her book became a best seller. It was a story of her successful conquest of dependency on alcohol.

"If you bring forth what is within you, it will save you. If you do not bring forth what is within you, it will destroy you,"[22] states St. Thomas in Gnostic writings. He confirms the biblical statement that "good men out of good treasures of the heart bring forth good things."[23]

Positive thinking is a matter of decision, but to acquire it requires practice and reinforcement of new beliefs by such activities as

- giving up obsolete beliefs that aging is hopeless and unavoidable;
- giving up the resistance to feel love, hope, and compassion for ourselves and others;
- avoiding relationships that pollute life;

- accepting responsibility for aging, thus controlling one's destiny;
- giving meaning to past or present pains, for there is a meaning in any suffering;
- living in the present with an awareness of tomorrow.

Reading of spiritual literature, listening to music or an inspirational speaker, practicing faith or a philosophical belief, and connecting with nature are means that sublimate forces that hold us back and contribute to the development of new beliefs about aging.

While our contributions to the immensity of the physical world appear to be minimal, our presence in the universe is of unimaginable significance. We, people, give meaning to the universe. Our presence is a reason great enough to justify its existence. And the fact that we are not a static, aimlessly procreating species, but we are changing, evolving, and directing the future of the world is essential for the new possibilities for humankind.

Viktor E. Frankl wrote in his best seller, *Man's Search for Meaning*, "that one cannot force oneself to be an optimist against all hope...as faith and love cannot be ordered."[24] There must be a reason for happiness. Once the reason is found, one becomes happy automatically. "People have enough to live but nothing to live for. They have the means but not the meaning."[25]

How does a human being go about finding the meaning? One has to create work or do a deed. In Frankl's words, "man should not ask what is the meaning of life but rather what is my potential and by finding it, bring it to fruition."[26]

The search for individual potential is endless for each of us uses only a very small part of it. To perceive oneself as a creation in the process of becoming opens doors to new horizons that can give any person not only new meaning and fulfillment, but can regenerate one's youth and vigor.

The Fountain of Energy

Nothing happens, unless something moves

—Albert Einstein[1]

Energy! Its power is vital for the activities of our bodies as well as for the motion of stellar bodies in the universe. Without energy, there would be no life as we know it.

Lack of energy is one of the most common complaints among seniors; therefore, it is crucial to understand where energy comes from, how to increase it, manage it, and preserve it for essential tasks and functions, particularly in later years of life when vitality tends to decline.

Human energy is a broad field, too complex to be elaborated on in detail, but even a partial glimpse on its salient features will be helpful in mastering its power to our benefit. The greater the awareness of energy, the more available it will be.

What is energy? Where does it come from? Can our bodies amplify it?

Before we unlock the access to the sources of higher energy, let us turn our attention to the bioenergetics and consumption of food, on which depends our bodies' survival. The energy that nourishes most of the world population emanates, to a great extent, from solar light, which some organisms are capable of converting into chemical energy into the form of organic molecules. This process, known as photosynthesis, produces a green molecule—chlorophyll. The energy from solar light merges with carbon dioxide and water and produces oxygen and organic matter that is known as the biomolecule glucose—a source of food that sustains us.

Our primary energy is derived from the food we eat. The human body burns it, metabolizes it into sugar, and transports it, in the form of glucose, to our cells. The quality and quantity of food we metabolize is measured by units representing amounts of energy—calories. The energy derived from food is channeled to support the kidneys, the heart, digestive organs, brain cells, or other vital functions such as the immune, endocrinal, and nervous systems. We know that individuals who are deprived of food for several days become weaker and after their organisms use all the bodily reserves, they die.

Depending on individual choices and needs, we consume about 60,000 to 100,000 pounds of food in our lifetimes.[2] Energy is produced by the transformation of the entering food through the biological "machines" in our cells that process it. Such machinery generates and carries energy from one place to another. The fascinating aspect of these biological machines is that they are extremely small, yet they efficiently work on micromolecular levels within the confines of every single cell. In that cell, so small that we cannot see it with the bare eye, biological energy is produced not by one, but thousands of identical machines, arranged in parallels and series, within each cellular organelle. The transducing element in each machine is a micromolecule that is in charge of delivering a specific chemical to the place where it belongs, for example, rhodopsin to the retina of the eye, or actomyosin to the muscles.

The glimpse into this very complex system of a microuniverse is helping us understand the importance of the food we eat. If we do not supply proper nutrients to specific areas of the body, such deprived parts will weaken and decline. On the other hand, if we eat nutrients obstructing the processing machinery in our biosystems, such as food loaded with cholesterol, our bodies will become clogged streams. The calls for help from our organisms are evident as symptoms: Whenever we have pain, high blood pressure, or some of our organs strike, we need to consider that our biological machinery is in need of repair.

We cannot preserve youth and vigor if we are misusing our bodies, decreasing their energy by improper diets, and, what is equally important, living without awareness that our bodies are gradually dying, due to neglect. Diabetes, heart disease, and emphysema are some of the examples of slow death of our organisms.

The importance of nutrition cannot be underestimated. Chapter 7 has been dedicated to enhancing our understanding of the food we eat and its impact on youth, vigor, and health.

■ ■ ■

There is yet another type of energy: Einstein's formulations of the energy-matter equation led to a postulation that mass and energy are interconvertible. Therefore, a constant transformation of matter into energy takes place, and vice versa. Food changes into energy through biological processes, and a similar transformation of energy and matter takes place in the universe on the thermonuclear level. Since vibrations of the universe are permeating our bodies, we are connected to the universal source of energy, even though we are not aware of it. While the connectedness with the universal energy and intelligence allows us to transcend our corporal boundaries and access higher energy, the bioenergy provides the needed supplies to our bodies to keep them alive. But how can we access the higher energy?

Astrophysicists accumulated facts in exploration of the universe by sophisticated telescopes of all lengths, radio waves, gamma rays, and other means, which allowed them to measure and to study objects as far as several billion light-years away. They found that some of the stellar bodies are older than our solar system itself. These observations have revealed a very complex universe where an intelligent energy maintains the planets pursuing their trajectories with atomic precision, controls the space temperature at such a level that the universe does not over-heat by billions of stars, and is kept in an immeasurable coordination.

We people gravitate to our planet, and our perception of reality is earthbound. We find it rather superfluous to give thoughts to the fact that the universe is filled with the same vibrations that make up the human body, albeit in a different density.[3]

Besides understanding the material aspects of the body's energy, it is essential to be aware of our connectedness with the universal energy of which we are an inseparable part. But what is universal energy?

■ ■ ■

Before the creation of the universe, according to astrophysicists, there was an infinite ether without a beginning or end. It was a timeless void destined to never change, never reinvent itself. St. Augustine described it as "The never ending present," thus conveying that time did not exist before creation.[4]

How did the universe come into being?

One of the first attempts to answer this eternal dilemma comes from the ancient philosopher Democritus who stated in the third century B.C. that "in the void, everything is in constant motion."[5] Aristotle called the ultimate energy Primum Mobile—the unmoved cosmos—from which all motions originate. Two millennia later, quantum physicists informed us that in the subatomic world nothing stands still—everything fluctuates.

It was believed that the universe was static until the beginning of the twentieth century, when a cosmologist, George Lemaître, observed that the galaxies were moving apart, that the universe was continually expanding. His observations were confirmed in 1948 by Edwin Hubble, who, with the help of his groundbreaking telescope, recorded that galaxies were indeed moving millions of miles per minute farther from each other. The discovery that the universe is inflating had far-reaching consequences. When the trajectories of the galaxies were reversed and followed to the point of their origin, it was evident that 14 billion years ago, they were compressed to an unimaginable density. The concentration of energy was equivalent to billions of galaxies compressed into a space smaller than the primal atom, to a point of infinite density of energy that led to the nuclear explosion of unimaginable proportion: to the beginning of our universe—the Big Bang.

As the cosmological expansion of the universe, after the Big Bang, was continuing, its temperature decreased below 1 thousand billion degrees; the radiation became less energetic until it was no longer strong enough to prevent nuclear bonding. The energy was diminishing, and stars died when they ran out of nuclear fuel. Without the energy of thermonuclear fusion, they could no longer support their weight and began to fade and collapse. What happened to the corpses and energy left from the stars? The recent astronomical community is accepting the explanation that black holes in the galaxies are the final disposal of corpses from the catastrophic death of massive stars.

German physicist Hermann von Helmholtz developed an analogy between the dying universe running down the way humans do. He called the process of slowdown and decay *entropy*—which meant that the energy of the universe was becoming less dense as time went by, until all the energy, one day, would be evenly distributed over the space and lead to the universe's ultimate end.

While the word entropy is frequently used in relation to an organism's slowdown due to time, Helmholtz's prophecy of inevitable progression of disorganization toward the decay and end of the universe took a surprising development. He built his assumptions on the second law of thermodynamics, stating that isolated systems cannot exchange energy with each other and become disorganized as time goes by.

But the universe is much more complex and unpredictable than Helmholtz thought. In 1998 two groups of astronomers[6] discovered that the universe is not slowing down, but is rather accelerating its expansion.

From what sources of energy was the sudden acceleration propelled?

Calculations indicated that there are two types of energy, not only one. Besides energy of motion, or kinetic energy, there is also stored energy, or potential energy. To simplify a very complex process, when the kinetic expansion was slowing down, and it was anticipated that it could reach a critical level of density leading to the destruction of life, the stored energy plugged in and started to accelerate the speed of universal expansion.[7]

It is awesome to realize that acceleration of the expansion took place some 5 billion years ago at a time when slowdown was anticipated to reach critical proportions, leading to the universe's ultimate entropy and end.

If the universe is so minutely coordinated, what intelligence is organizing it and for what purpose? Our existence down here is not as insignificant as it might appear, but from an eternal perspective, has a higher meaning, that we, humans, try to understand through scientific explorations or to accept through faith.

The infinite energy of our universe is an inspiring analogy, showing us the way to the source of our own hidden energy. The question we have to ask is, from where did the energy originate that accelerated the expansion of our universe at a critical time?

Professor Marcelo Gleiser concludes ongoing research in his book, *The Prophet and the Astronomer,* by suggesting that energy came from cosmic voids, or empty spaces, of the universe that are filled with dark energy of enormous power.[8] Calculations indicate that dark matter contributes about 70 percent of the critical density of the universe.[9]

It means that the future of the universe depends on the mysterious invisible voids filled with dark energy.

There is not yet a particle physics model that can explain such phenomena. All we know is that the mysterious energy did set in when there was a need for an extraordinary intervention: saving the universe from the anticipated "crunch" and destruction.

As the universe is expanding, so are we. From year to year we change and expand toward new goals, while solving problems, and discovering new aspects of ourselves in fulfilling our purpose down here.

If the body is a microcosm of the universe, would it be possible that we, too, have the "empty spaces" of energy that can be released under special circumstances? Do we have evidence that a dormant, unsuspected potential is waiting in us for an opportunity to be used for a vital purpose?

The mysterious source of energy supporting life under the most traumatic circumstances was manifested in the writing of Viktor E. Frankl, survivor of several concentration camps, in his book *Man's Search for Meaning*. In spite of inhumane conditions at the barracks, he was performing the most demanding manual tasks, such as digging frozen ground and laying tracks for the railroad line, in freezing weather, or taking care of patients in the typhus ward. Every day, regardless of fever, illness, edema, frostbitten feet, and physical weakness due to a lack of food and hunger, he was ready to work because whoever did not report for work in the morning was sent to a gas chamber.[10] Frankl survived this ordeal for many years. The question of how he could possibly endure this extraordinary hardship when so many others gave up is a manifestation of the powerful field of energy he was able to connect with regardless of physical conditions. His purpose to survive was a bridge connecting him to sources of energy that cannot be explained by bioenergetics alone, but suggests access to a higher power that he tapped by transcending the physical self.

If we are convinced that life here serves a purpose and human energy is dedicated to the fulfillment of that purpose, we are able to overcome most difficult obstacles. The spiritual energy supports us in the most difficult circumstances and transforms us toward ever new levels of "humanness" rather than pulling us toward despair, decay, and entropy.

▨ ▨ ▨

Einstein equated matter to stored energy. His famous equation, $E = mc^2$, means that under the proper circumstances, matter can change into energy of an equivalent amount to that matter. Nothing, not even an atom, gets lost in the universe.[11] Thus, the energy invested into human actions also is expected to be transformed into something of equivalent value.

If we think of humans as being part of the cosmic "soup" where protons, neutrons, and electrons are roaming the universe with light-weight particles such as quarks, leptons, photons, gravitons, hadrons, neutrinos, and tau among others, we realize that we are part of an immense energy field that is available to us, not physically, but through our conscious connection with it.

Joseph Campbell supports this perception of higher energy: "There is consciousness in the body. The whole living world is informed by consciousness. I have a feeling that consciousness and energy are the same thing...Where you see life energy, there is consciousness."[12]

Consciousness of organisms was recognized in the thirteenth century by St. Thomas Aquinas, when he stated that each element in nature directs itself toward the fulfillment of its function.[13] Exploration of the universal energy attracted many scientists, too numerous to be mentioned here. Among them was the French physician Dr. Hyppolyte Baraduc, who called energy the vital force, and a noted phenomenologist, Pierre Teilhard de Chardin, stating that universal energy is thinking energy.

We all have access to this conscious energy that can work for us, if we are aware of it and learn how to connect with its intelligence.

When we want to purchase a car, a house, or make any other financial investment, we give considerable thought to what is the best deal and explore alternatives to get the maximum value for our cash before making a commitment.

When investing our energies, we are much less concerned with what we are getting in return. If we are spending our material assets with such caution, why are we much less concerned with what we are getting for investing our energies? Frequently, we misinvest our precious powers, which can make us emotionally exhausted or bankrupt. An awareness of how to spend energy, particularly in the later years of life, is vital if we want to stay vigorous, independent, and healthy.

How can we save and amplify energy? It is not of general knowledge that the daily ratio of energy must go somewhere, since we cannot save it by being inactive. If we do not invest it constructively, or if we do not spend it at all, it will discharge itself destructively. Horney pointed out that man's essential nature is in the constructive possibilities of his core. Man turns unconstructive and destructive only if he cannot fulfill himself.

Any activity that fulfills one with the sense of purpose, meaning, self-esteem, or well-being is a well-spent energy that replenishes itself and amplifies one's vigor.[14]

If we use energy on obsessing about past events, feeling guilty, worrying excessively, hating someone, replaying traumatic events of the past, or being stuck in another kind of mental rumination, we are discharging our precious power destructively. Such activities lead to tiredness, lack of fulfillment, exhaustion, and loss of vigor. Dr. Deepak Chopra states in his book *Ageless Body, Timeless Mind* that remembering stress releases the same flood of destructive hormones as the stress itself.[15] Because the mind influences every cell in the body, the energy we spend on gossip, idle talk, chronic arguments, and wasteful acting out turns into a negative force such as depressed mood, irritability, insomnia, unhappiness, emptiness, or other negative emotions. In his book *Core Energetics*, Dr. John C. Pierrakos presents the idea that destructive thoughts block free flow of energy and prevent us from healing.[16] Access to our energy can be unlocked when we overcome mechanistic, unconscious actions and thoughts and plug into our conscious, creative energy.

Dimitri de Berea, the last student of Professor Pierre Bonnard, who himself became a noted portraitist of European aristocracy, revealed how difficult it was to balance his physical and creative energies. While starting a portrait in 1966, he said,

> I find it very difficult to face the day in the morning. I feel tired when I awake, wishing I would not have to get up and work. What triggers my energy is the thought that I have a painting on the easel. When I begin to think about it, suddenly something clicks in my mind: Inspiration! I begin to imagine, for example, what color I would use for a particular detail and before I know it, I get off my bed and rush to my studio, often skipping breakfast, eager to try something new. I become so immersed in painting that sometimes I work until noon or later without noticing that

time is passing. I experience elation and fulfillment…a peak creative experience. After such spontaneous work, I do not feel tired or hungry, on the contrary, I am invigorated by my work.[17]

New streams of ideas that spring into existence from a source within our field of awareness is not diminishing energy, but rather producing greater accomplishments with less expenditure of energy than the automatic behavior.

Activities that exhaust energy should be avoided. Relationships that pollute life are not only obnoxious to our psychological health, they absorb an exorbitant amount of energy.

Stress has a detrimental effect on body and mind. It depletes energy faster than a full day of work. Moreover, it contributes to illness, aging, and entropy. Stress can be avoided if we redefine the problem and reinvent ourselves accordingly. When old beliefs and attitudes no longer work for us, we have to look for new ways to deal with stressful situations. Our decisions to become aware of stress triggers will create an immediate reaction in our biochemical responses and inspire us to elevate ourselves to a different level of understanding. We cannot defeat entropy as a physical force; we can only elevate ourselves above it to a spiritual level where entropy cannot reach us.

What can we do to increase our energy levels?

The first step starts with giving up the obsolete belief that loss of energy is caused by aging. Such assumptions are, for the most part, misleading because any person, young or old, can experience loss of energy for various reasons other than age. To anticipate that energy will decline with chronological age is to program ourselves for failure.

Second, we cannot become aware of energy unless we decide to make a commitment to it. The connectedness will not happen automatically. There are billions of impulses per minute in our brains that interact and distract us from using energy consciously, unless we practice self-awareness.

Third, whenever we give our energies to a person or a cause, we have to do it from the position of generosity and power. If we are giving energy against our wills, such gifts do not empower us, but weaken and impoverish us. It is awareness of our powers to give that is a life-changing experience, elevating us above material concerns and replenishing energy we spent.

There are many ways to save energy; among them is the practice of meditation, various types of yoga, or any other spiritual exercises that calm the mind and induce a state of relaxation. Conscious energy management results in reduced levels of cortisol and adrenaline, also lowers the blood pressure, breathing intensity, and heartbeat. The power of spiritual practice and concentration prevents the scattering of thoughts into irrelevant and wasteful venues, thus liberating energy for actions that count. Yoga Nidra, which means "sleep," is particularly helpful for the induction of relaxation.

One of the helpful techniques to unclutter life from wasteful thoughts is the practice of mandala. Mandala is the Sanskrit word for circle. You may imagine an invisible circle around your body, or you may actually draw one in the sand on the beach or by chalk on your carpet or floor. Sitting in the middle of the mandala helps to concentrate on issues that are of value to you, to pull together those fragmented aspects of life. While sitting in the circle, you may think of your connectedness with the universal energy of which you are a part, and, by doing so, come to the empowering feeling that you are the center of your world. Where you are, there is peace and order. Practice of mandala focuses attention and concentration and results in an amplification of vital energy and a sense of personal power.

To dedicate 20–30 minutes daily to silence is another powerful means to save energy. We are surrounded by environmental noises, originating from city, nature, household, and workplace sources. Our brain consists of 100 billion neurons that on the unconscious level process 400 billion bits of information per minute, or a thousand trillion synapses. Daily commitment to a "time of silence" can save considerable energy spent on reacting to irrelevant stimuli. To reduce irritable interference, use of an eye mask or earplugs may protect us from distraction. Settled in a comfortable position, in a quiet room, with reduced lights and closed eyes, we may imagine ourselves being far away at a peaceful location, whether it be a distant island, a mountaintop, or any other fantasy of your choice. Or, we may take a power nap and disconnect from thoughts and noises.

Dr. Joan LaMontagne, psychologist and writer, suggests recognition of the wavelike activity of sequences of rest and action throughout the day. The trigger for rest is the satisfaction of a job well done or a sign of tiredness or inefficiency for some. To take a "power nap" regenerates energy and energizes conscious activities.[18]

To perpetuate a youthful vigor, we have to elevate ourselves above time, dependency, negative thoughts, and physical limitations. The intention to actualize our innate gifts and talents is sometimes as good as if we already achieved a higher spiritual standing. It is the commitment to greater wholeness and humanness that counts. However, the source of energy and creativeness is available only in response to a genuine interest in it. The effort to explore the other aspects of being means that one has to get to its deeper layers with a determination and a sense of curiousity.

Those seniors who committed themselves to new frontiers of aging through self-actualization are, according to Maslow, more efficient, happy, serene, wise, better organizers and perceivers, and it is easier for them to make decisions.[19]

To seek new experiences of aging through our vocations, interests, desires, and needs fulfill us. The realization of the difference between mechanical, unconscious existence versus living our destinies fills us with a profound conviction that we are on the "right track." The awareness that energy serves activities that are returning it back to its universal source may lead to a spiritual climax that renews vigor and regenerates us in future endeavors.

■ ■ ■

According to astrophysicists, we are stardust. "The chemistry of our bodies is derived from explosions that occurred well before the formation of our solar system," says Gleiser.[20] However, we are stardust with a consciousness. The latter asset enables us to live on higher than materialistic levels. It is the consciousness of ourselves that enables us to live above entropy and decay, using the higher energy, whether we call it spiritual or creative power, that propels us toward the realization of our unique potentials, giving ever-new meaning to our existence down here.

5 ▪ ▪ ▪

Changing Face of Love and Sensuality

"Omnia Vincit Amor"
Love conquers everything

—Virgil[1]

Love is ageless. It is a profound emotion that can be experienced by any person regardless of age, culture, or health status. It is a fundamental part of the real self and reveals itself in the most unexpected moments of life, even when we sometimes feel that we are emotionally dead.

The focus of this chapter is on the changing needs of the senior population in the sphere of love and sexuality. As seniors live longer and healthier lives, the available energy and libido are extending the possibility for intimate interaction until an advanced age. Many modern seniors are asking what is expected from them sexually as they age: Is it ethical to have sex in "old" age? Does aging affect erectile functions? Does menopause decrease the capacity for good sex?

While our knowledge about human sexuality has greatly increased since the studies of William H. Masters and Virginia E. Johnson,[2] much less is known about the frequency and the quality of sexuality in the later years of life. While some seniors continue to enjoy sex until an advanced age, others agree with the Greek poet Sophocles who, in his 80s, felt relieved from "the tyranny" of Venus—the goddess of love.[3]

The following review of the evolution of intimate relationships between men and women illustrates the long history of its constant transformation from lower to higher levels of humanity that still continues to evolve as we enter the third millennia. Seniors, living far beyond their personal and societal expectations, search for a new expression of human sexuality that would be in harmony with their extended life spans, moral and esthetic values, and their health statuses.

▦ ▦ ▦

Sexual contact between men and women can be traced to the beginning of humanity when *Homo sapiens* attempted to attract the best possible mate for procreation. The preference for partners can be observed even in studies of baboons in Africa, where some female baboons longed for their former male who was defeated by a stronger but less compatible rival. As the prefrontal cortex gradually evolved, people were able to think about their choices, and the need for greater compatibility increased.

During the first millennium A.D., marital unions were dominated by socioreligious values and arranged by families based on reason. It was only in the twelfth century when romantic love was finally publicly recognized. Troubadours were singing about an all-absorbing passion, or *Amor,* based on a special chemistry between two people. The famous story of Tristan and Isolde reflected the power of romantic love for which young people were willing to give up their lives. The deaths of Romeo and Juliet were the epitome of such a love. "Love is the high point of life. It is the meaning of life," stated Joseph Campbell.[4] Through love, individuals can experience eternity.

Besides *Amor* and *Eros,* which is a biological urge for sex, there is also *Agape,* or love born from compassion: "Love thy neighbor as you love thyself." This human emotion, extended to any person in the form of compassion, can also be experienced as friendship. Being a good friend by taking time to listen and respond with empathy represents a high level of exchange between two or more people who have a natural compatibility. Compassionate friendship, whether based on daily or occasional contact, is of particular importance to seniors who are often living far away from their children or relatives and stay involved with life through friends and social acquaintances.

The onset of the twentieth century brought the psychoanalytic movement that highlighted yet another type of relationship: *the attachment.* Attachment is the very early tie between mother and child that is expected to gradually decrease, resulting in the child's ability to become emotionally independent. However, if the separation is delayed or sometimes never resolved due to a mother's personality or other reasons, when the child becomes an adult, the attachment is transferred onto the partner. While the attachment, with its dependency, may appear as love, it is far from it.

In mature love, an individual is a free agent, able to give and receive love on the basis of emotional reciprocity. In attachment, a person is dependent on the other partner's availability and presence. One is not complete without the other person. When the spouse dies, the unresolved attachment is frequently transferred to the adult children or other relationships. We recognize such seniors by their need to lean on someone, often by their helplessness and inability to live alone, even though they are physically healthy. The difference between attachment and love is sometimes difficult to discern. In attachment, two people merge while diminishing their individual identities. In love, two people, who know each other's soul, remain independent.

Mrs. S., 72 years of age, was a textbook example of what happens to an attached person when she is abandoned. After 52 years in a childless marriage, filled with a shallow social life, her husband told her that he felt emotionally dead in her presence and cannot live with her anymore. He packed and went to Las Vegas where he had previously developed relationships with other women. Mrs. S. was both financially and emotionally dependent on her husband. Her attachment to him turned into despair: "How could he do this to me?" she asked in disbelief. Her shock turned into rage of abandonment when her husband asked for a divorce. Two years of therapy were not sufficient to reverse the attachment pattern. When she received a favorable financial settlement from her husband, she moved to Florida to a senior residence where her dependency on others continued. To overcome lifelong attachment requires desire for autonomy, determination, and hard work, skills that Mrs. S. persistently avoided.

British psychiatrist John Bowlby dedicated his professional career to the subject of attachment and loss. His work demonstrated that attachment comes from a need for security; therefore, the greater the attachment, the more devastating the loss.[5]

It is a joy when marriage or a committed relationship brings harmony and fulfillment to both partners. During the happy years, neither of the partners gives thought to the possibility that life could end. There is well-known resistance to plan for the inevitable moment of separation, even among the most informed and otherwise responsible individuals.

It was a shock when John Dunne, the husband of best-selling author Joan Didion, died. In her book, *The Year of Magical Thinking,* Didion remembers 40 years of togetherness during her marriage that suddenly ended. For all those years, she saw herself "through the eyes of her husband,"[6] and she was not aging. "Marriage was not only time passing, it was paradoxically a denial of time."[7] Then, her life suddenly changed: It changed fast, in an instant. She sat down to dinner, and life, as she knew it, ended. Her husband died at the dinner table following a stroke.

Whether the departed spouse was dearly loved or whether the relationship was tense, a resolution of the ties must follow. Grief and mourning are basic for a healthy adaptation to the loss. Reaction to death may include deep pain, emptiness, fear, or anger, depending on the circumstances. There is a sense of powerlessness regarding the loss, especially when illness, alcohol, deficient doctors and care, or a lack of cooperation from the deceased are to blame. When the death occurred after a long illness, the remaining spouse may experience relief after years of stress. A burnout is frequently a consequence of caring for a chronically ill family member.

Normal grief may extend to two years, but when mourning becomes a way of life, and the adjustment to a new life situation is not taking place, a depressive reaction may be the cause of the delay; a professional consultation should be sought to accelerate the process of recovery.

At other situations, the loss of a spouse is a trigger for change and development of personality features that were suppressed during the marriage. The incomplete development, which the remaining partner could not fulfill in the past, can now be reactivated. Interest in new pursuits accelerate the resolution of grief and starts a new phase of life focusing on different objectives, such as adult children, grandchildren, a return to work, or the consideration of a new partner. Adaptation to single life after the death of a spouse is more difficult for men than for women; statistics indicate that widowers have a higher rate of remarriage than widows do.

Even in the best marriages memories sometimes cause pain or resentment after the death of a spouse. The surviving partner has a choice: either to remember the pain and thus be forever attached to the past or to forgive and forget the pain and become free from it. Through anger, we are bound forever; through forgiveness, we receive the great reward of emotional freedom that opens doors to new vistas in life, intended for us by the universal design.

But not all marriages end by extended widowhood: Mr. and Mrs. B. celebrated their 50th anniversary together with their two sons, daughters-in-law, and several grandchildren, who came from distant parts of the country for the festive occasion.

Several weeks later, Mrs. B. awoke in the morning as usual and to the dismay of her husband said, "I know you, but I cannot remember your name." It was the beginning of a devastating discovery that she was suffering from dementia. Mr. B. took dedicated care of her as she was gradually losing touch with her environment. He declined help until a fateful winter night, when Mrs. B. got the uncontrollable idea that she was expected at a cocktail party. She attempted to get dressed, insisting to leave the house. Mr. B. was a rather frail man and found it difficult to restrain his wife. Only after this traumatic experience did Mr. B. consent to accept the help of a caretaker for a half-day. By doctor's order, he was directed to spend the other half of the day at a senior center, so that he may regain energy and regenerate his mind. But when he returned home, he could not wait to see his old life partner who intuitively waited for him. When they met, the joy in her eyes lit and warmed the heart of the old man. "I could not wait to see you, old girl," said Mr. B., and they embraced as in the old days. It was the priceless reward in spite of suffering the deterioration of the mind.

When the decline in both spouses could no longer be contained within the home environment, they were transferred to a nursing facility, but not for long. When Mrs. B. died of a stroke, her husband followed her several days later, while resting in a recliner and listening to ballroom music that they both had enjoyed in the past.

■ ■ ■

Seniors who remarry or date in later years have mixed emotions regarding sexuality, ranging from elation to caution. There are generational as well as personal reasons for such differences, including fear of failure, loyalty to a deceased partner, moral rationale that sex is only for procreation, concern about being disappointed, or a lack of information.

The popular saying "The lights are on, but the voltage is low" is, according to John W. Rowe and Robert L. Kahn, a myth rather than a reality.[8] Such statements express the "pluralistic ignorance" and fiction that chronological age is a factor in decreasing sexuality. Statistical evidence in Richard Schulz and Timothy Salthouse's *Adult Development and Aging* indicates that, according to longitudinal studies, the first substantial drop in sexual interest is noticed around the age of 50. At the age of 60, 53–80 percent of men are sexually active, at the age of 70, 45 percent are active, and at the age of 78, 25 percent are active.[9] Considering that the longitudinal studies were assessing data in the distant past, it can be anticipated that sexuality among seniors will increase due to longevity and better health. However, it is not age but hormonal changes, poor health, stress, overwork, and the loss of a partner that are the leading causes of a decrease in sexual activity. Moreover, new evidence stresses that lack of exercise, unhealthy diet, and poor nutrition also contribute to reduced health and libido.

There is no scientific evidence that menopause decreases interest in sexual activity in women. While the frequency of sex in healthy women is a matter of individual choice, there is a significant decrease of activity following the loss of a spouse. Studies indicate that women who enjoyed sex during their youth and marriage will be sexually active longer than women who were less interested in sex.

In general, men and women do not change much in their patterns of intimate relationships developed during adulthood and marriage. Those who had consistent sexual experiences in the past continue to be sexually active until an advanced age. The concept of "use it or lose it" is applicable to all physical and mental functions, including sex. The determining factor is physical health. Oxygen use during sexual activity and orgasm is equivalent to climbing a flight of stairs or walking briskly for 15 minutes.

Most of the recent studies highlight the importance of orgasm as a contributing factor to healthy arteries, reduced stress level, better sleeping habits, and lower blood pressure. A well-known study done in 1950 by Duke University researchers indicated that frequency and enjoyment of sex is correlated with longevity.[10]

With increasing numbers of seniors using such libido boosters as Cialis and Levitra, voices of concern can be heard as to the side effects of such hormones on health. Medical consultation before the use of such products should be obligatory.

We have to be careful not to be misled by our egos, or libido-boosting publicity, which attempt to convince us that seniors have boundless energy that can be indiscriminately invested into sex, new relationships, and projects at no cost. The truth is that energy has to be budgeted so that it is invested in activities that energize, but do not exhaust us. If seniors feel that sex or relationships, instead of being enjoyable, are increasingly draining on energy, then a decision to change is in order. The couple will benefit by jointly exploring alternatives that would be acceptable to both of them. For love without truth and truth without freedom are not possible. It is difficult to love another if we cannot love ourselves. Seniors must love and respect their own bodies first. To please a partner and suppress our own needs is not love. It leads to poor self-esteem, anger, and alienation. One of the great advantages of the mature years is the wisdom to recognize that we have needs and that they have to be met in order for us to care for others. Awareness and reverence for our bodies are paths leading to self-respect, generosity, mutual understanding, and fulfillment.

▪ ▪ ▪

Research indicates that with advancing years, the differences in seniors' lifestyles, appearances, health, and sexuality deepens. It is unfortunate when different paces of aging takes place in a marriage: One partner keeps young and vigorous and the other gives into the lower self and entropy. Lasting relationships do not depend on sex, but more so on emotional compatibility and common goals that bind two people together. Regardless of age, love is hard work that requires self-discipline, commitment to the higher self, adaptability to changing circumstances, and respect for the partner. When two people can exchange positive energy with each other, it ultimately leads to a unifying experience and love. Exchanging negative energy results in hurt, disappointment, and distancing. Positive forces include kindness, tolerance, or support, and negative energy is criticism, resentment, impatience, and ignorance. A relationship requires commitment, and the partners must decide on priorities for investing their energies into mutually acceptable objectives.

People of all ages fall in love. J. Howard Marshall, 89 years old, married a much younger Anna Nicole Smith; Charlie Chaplin, in his mid-50s, fell in love with Oona O'Neil, and they had eight children, the last of which was born when he was 72 years of age. A 60-year-old woman recently gave birth to a child, fathered by a younger man, an event making headlines in several newspapers in 2007. There are thousands of relationships and marriages where men and women of advanced age find the love of their lives in later years.

There is no consensus on what it means to "fall in love." However, John C. Pierrakos elaborates in the book *Eros, Love & Sexuality* on an irresistible attraction that two people may suddenly feel without knowing one another.[11] The attraction—or Eros—can disappear as fast as it appeared, leaving behind disappointment and sometimes causing depressive reactions. On the other hand, Eros can become a basis on which to build a loving relationship, provided that both parties are committed to do the hard work required of such a union.

Dr. Helen E. Fisher used neurophysiological research to explore the love connection in relation to brain chemistry. She wanted to know what causes the urge to desire another person. Her findings have implications for seniors as well. What Homer called the "pulsing rush of longing"[12] is, according to Fisher, a chemical reaction in the prefrontal cortex of the brain to mate.

From a biological perspective, the prefrontal cortex, located behind the forehead, is collecting data from our senses, evaluates and integrates them, makes choices, and controls our basic drives. It is this part of the brain that reasons, deliberates, and decides on the choice of our partner. One part of the prefrontal cortex, the caudate nucleus, fuels passion by increasing the emission of the neurotransmitter dopamine that regulates emotions, releases testosterone, and promotes sexual activity. Those who have higher levels of testosterone tend to engage in sex more readily than do those with lower levels. "We are built to love at any age," states Fisher. "Men and women in their seventies, eighties, even nineties, also feel a love...a study of 225 adolescents, young adults, middle-aged men and women and senior citizens found no overall difference in the intensity of their romantic passion."[13]

It is mostly a myth that age is a determining factor in sexual performance and capacity to love. Plasticity of the prefrontal cortex and other vital organs and a suitable partner are the stimulating triggers that lead to the release of dopamine, desire, and intimate activities. The frequency and degree of passion and vigor may fluctuate with the change of circumstances and new opportunities: An attractive editor complained of impotency since he was 60 years of age, but developed a passionate affair at the age of 82 with a sexual intensity unparalleled in his prior life.

There is not one definition of love or sex. Nevertheless, it is rather self-evident that relationships that are exploitative, where partners have hidden agendas, where it is always questionable who controls whom, and who is right or wrong, lead to stress and unhappiness. On the other hand, when two people have arranged their relationship in such a way that one person's advantage is to the other person's benefit also, then the couple can meet and master the problems of life and enrich each other in a great way.

A long-standing relationship can be a source of great enjoyment or of distress. Marriage can drain vitality and aliveness if it is not revived as time passes by. Those who reached a critical level of enmeshment might need to practice disengagement from the marital dyad. The more one leans on a partner, the greater the likelihood to become gradually helpless. And helplessness is a learned habit that may lead to a loss of independence. If both partners can see the advantage of creative living by regenerating themselves individually as well as reinventing their relationship, they may discover new aspects of marriage never experienced before. Peak experiences are possible if there is a burning desire for problem solving and commitment to each other.

What is needed to sustain a relationship in later years?

From several studies dealing with regeneration of relationships, we would suggest the following steps:

- **Power of positive thinking:** All problems have solutions: to think creatively is a positive approach, to follow old habits leads to patterned living, which reduces the capacity for problem solving.
- **Open communication:** Do not assume that you know your partner. People change, and their needs and choices change with them. Do not deprive your partner of the freedom to express the most private wishes by guessing his or her thoughts; ask and expect answers.

- **Metabolizing disappointments:** Broken promises, forgotten anniversaries, lingering illness, unexpected financial problems, and canceled vacations all tend to spoil anticipated joy. How you perceive the disappointment can make a difference. Nobody can hurt or disappoint you without your permission.

- **Manage space and involvement:** Space in advanced years is essential for creative living, particularly if your quarters are not spacious. To create space, discuss a division of areas that you need for essential activities. Negotiate on days when you will spend time with family or friends. If you are suffocating in an environment that is too small for you, get a job, go back to college, volunteer, babysit for your grandchildren, but do not sit at home and complain.

- **Quality versus quantity:** It is not necessarily the quantity of time spent together that counts, but also the quality of time spent away from each other that adds to marital enrichment and variety. The statement that love conquers everything is a daily crucible, testing the depth of commitment to the marriage.

- **Emerging differences:** As spouses are changing throughout years of life together, they may realize one day that the partner's characteristics that they admired in the past are gone, and some unwanted habits took their places. The most painful moment is the realization that one is no longer appreciated. At such moments, avoid frivolous decisions and reach toward the greatness of the real self for solutions, wisdom, and objectivity. Through creative alternatives, a relationship can be elevated to superior levels of understanding and acceptance. Professional help is sometimes, but not always, needed.

- **Decisive moments:** If you become emotionally disconnected from your spouse, or bored with each other, or if there is a third person in the picture, do not wait. Ask a recognized marriage therapist to assess the situation and develop alternatives. The ability to change and the capacity to love are two powerful allies in marital transformation. You cannot control unexpected events in life, but you have choices.

If your relationship does not improve by your own efforts, and you resist professional help, read at least some of the inspirational books that will help you to solve your situation creatively. Dr. Phillip C. McGraw's best-seller *Relationship Rescue*[14] and Dr. Aaron T. Beck's *Love Is Never Enough*[15] offer helpful ideas for renewal of lasting relationships.

▨ ▨ ▨

In addition to love and sex, there is a broad field of nonverbal interaction: It is the invaluable importance of the human touch. The need for it is as old as humanity. It is the most developed sensory modality at birth and contributes to cognitive and socioemotional development throughout childhood. Age does not diminish the need for touching as a means of communication and remains a vital part of contact with the environment.

Tactile contact can express not only erotic feelings, but also anger, hostility, aggression, or other negative emotions. But its prevalent value is in communicating positive feelings of affection, gratitude, caring, love, support, and an infinite variety of more subtle emotions. Its healing qualities are demonstrated by numerous studies.

Every person has about 75 trillion cells in his or her body. Each cell is equipped with sensors that not only receive information, but also process them and thus influence genes and brain activity. If the signal is negative, the brain and cells act to protect the organism. If the message is positive and pleasurable, the brain informs cells to relax, enjoy, and revitalize.

One of the most common ways of touching is contact by the lips. A kiss is a universal symbol of intimacy, affection, lust, and of an almost infinite range of other emotions. Whether it is a maternal kiss to a child, an apostolic "holy" kiss as a sign of agape, a marital kiss as a symbol of union, a passionate kiss between lovers, or a friendly kiss among relatives and friends, kiss plays an important role throughout life. Its execution varies, but the emotional range survives decades. A heart-to-heart kiss can trigger a firework of affection in the lonely heart of a man or woman, young or old.

While any person can communicate emotions through touch, there are specific criteria for therapeutic touching, such as medical massage or healing touch. In the early 1980s, Dr. John Zimmerman completed studies on therapeutic touch at the University of Colorado, School of Medicine in Denver, which recorded biomagnetic pulsation from the hands of the same wave frequencies as those of the brain, able to stimulate healing in any part of the body.[16] Healing touch is part of the holistic practice based on what Hypocrites called "the vital spirit," Chinese physicians call "chi," and the Hindus "prana." Diane W. Wardell, RNC, Ph.D., professor at the University of Texas, and Kathryn F. Weymouth, Ph.D., state that "the principle of the work of the body is a complex energy system that can be affected by another system to promote well-being. It includes the intention and placement of hands on specific areas of the body."[17] Other professionals, such as M.P. Fields, Ph.D., point to the benefits of the human touch by professional massage. Healing touch is currently a complementary therapy that is provided by nurses under the National Health Center for Complementary and Alternative Medicine of the National Institutes of Health. It is a biofeedback or energy-based therapy, a practice that is becoming increasingly prevalent.

Christiane Northrup, M.D., states that skin is a receptor of messages from the environment, such as temperature, meteorological pressure, ultraviolet rays, air pollution, or bacteria and viruses.[18] Dermatologists know that there is a connection between healthy skin, emotions, and the mind. Dermatitis and hives are examples of physical conditions that are psychologically affected and manifested through the skin.

Ellen K. Torronto, Ph.D., sees a reactivation of empathetic attunement in the human touch, a place of holding that allows the child a safe place for development. This "holding environment" can be of vital importance to seniors, particularly at a time of illness, loss of a spouse, or other change they may be facing. Physical touch may send a unique kind of soothing message to the organism, which is difficult to utter by verbal means only.[19]

Everyone needs physical reassurance from time to time, especially when facing pressures for constant adaptation to changing environments. In the absence of physical touch, we become emotionally isolated, lonely, and even self-esteem may gradually diminish. Human touch not only communicates an interpersonal connection, but it also increases our energy and well-being.

Who will hug or touch us lovingly when our spouses are no longer with us, when our children are often living far away, or when some of our friends lose their abilities for touching and are suppressing the need for affection?

Dr. Wardell and Dr. Weymouth reported in their studies of "Review of Studies of Healing Touch" that besides reduced pain, mental clarity, improved posture, and other physical improvements, healing touch massages also improve mood, well-being, interpersonal relationships, increase vitality, and decrease fatigue and blood pressure. In a controlled study of the elderly, C. Gehlhaart and P. Dail reported significant improvements in sleep, appetite, freedom from pain, orientation, socialization, emotional stability, and verbal communication.[20]

While it is difficult to replace the personal hug of a close person, it is in the best interest of an individual's health to find alternatives for the human touch. Without physical contact, we deprive ourselves of the vital experiences that keep our emotional, nonverbal dialogue with the environment alive. The skilled hands of a trained, caring professional convey to our bodies and minds that we are not isolated entities, but are a part of a vibrant interaction between caring people and the energy of the universe.

In the absence of a partner, family members, or friends to meet the need for human touch, professional help is just a telephone call away. What are we waiting for?

■ ■ ■

We are defined by what we desire most. It is possible to experience love, sex, affection and friendship, or peak experiences regardless of age because what determines the fulfillment of our objectives are our beliefs, lifestyle, strength of our desire, commitment, and perseverance—not our ages. The uniqueness of the real self helps to shape the individual's vision of love and sex throughout life, regardless of age because it is inspired by sources beyond our full control.

Do we ever quit hoping for love? "Dum spiro-spero," was the favored answer of poets in antiquity. "As long as we breath, we hope."

6 ▪ ▪ ▪

The Creative Process of Life

Give me the courage, Almighty to move forward when I would like
to stand still.

—[Anonymous prayer]

In the context of extended longevity, the 65th birthday is considered
the end of middle age. Whether we plan to retire at the age of 60, 70,
later, or never, we have to take a realistic look at our futures and visual-
ize where we want to be personally, professionally, and socially in the
next 10, 20, or 30 years.

The end of middle age is an occasion for reevaluation of past events,
review of personal inventory, and decision making regarding the future.
Certain common events impact life and set the stage for change. These
events include, but are not limited to, the following:

- retirement and reevaluation of professional goals;
- changes in family constellation due to empty nest syndrome, death, major
  illness, or divorce;
- changes in health: the bodies that served us for many decades—in some
  cases, in spite of the excessive use or consumption of alcohol, food, drugs,
  or smoking—start showing signs of wear and tear and call for attention
  and change in lifestyle;
- a review of life achievements, which reminds us of missed opportunities in
  the past, renews a desire to give old dreams another chance.

Everybody wants to age successfully, but what, after all, does it mean, to age successfully? seniors ask.

Aging successfully is a personal experience, something you desire, plan for, and work toward; it is the difference between health and illness, independence and dependency, productivity and passivity, generativity[1] and despair, a life of purpose and a life of doubts, and agelessness versus imitation of youth. If we want to age successfully, it will not happen because we have good genes, but rather it will be a result of our choices and work. Noted author and philosopher José Ortega y Gasset stated that in order to make decisions, we must have definite ideas about what to do.[2]

Do you have "definite ideas" about your future?

The better we can forecast our futures, the more in control we are about our destinies and success.

Average Americans spend one-third of their lives in retirement, according to sociologist Mathilde Riley.[3] The question is what to do with this one-third of life and to not waste it. Modern seniors have unique opportunities to start this new and exciting stage of life because they have wisdom, experience, time, and means to accomplish something they always wanted to do, and to reinvent themselves. But do they have the courage to consider change?

Whether we are aware of it or not, life is a constant process of change. We need to look for new solutions in the rise of daily challenges and to interpret them in different ways than we did in the past. It would be a delusion to believe that we can sustain a status quo—a state of no change—by living according to the old habits that we developed in the past. Patterns of life "as usual" undermine the renewal of our minds and bodies: Old solutions no longer work for us as we are developing and changing to a new worldview and perception of ourselves, not as aging, but as discovering new aspects of life.

We cannot stop the natural process of life that imposes on us constant change, but we can influence how to change and whom we want to become. While living by habits leads to inertia and mindlessness, accepting change as means of renewal allows for new possibilities that point to more abundant energy, alternatives, and fulfillment.

To define our future in the sixth or seventh decade of life can be as exciting or perplexing as was the decision making during college years. The search for new interests and goals can be exhilarating for some, while confusing for others. Results of recent research confirm that the further we go, the greater are the differences among seniors in their independence, appearances, health, and activities. The older we grow, the more choices we have to develop our unique potentials, to improve our lifestyles, and to extend our independence.

Literature by such spiritual authors as Viktor E. Frankl, Abraham H. Maslow, Joseph Campbell, Deepak Chopra, and others points to inspiring evidence that life can be greatly enhanced and transformed into an experience far beyond our expectations if we transcend the limitations of the physical body, develop a vision of the future, are conscious of all possibilities, and believe in our potentials. While this chapter is a roadmap to creative living, some seniors find it difficult to give up old beliefs that aging is a process of unavoidable decline, ending in loss of autonomy and death.

I frequently hear participants in my public appearances ask, "I worked for many years. Do I not deserve rest and time for leisure?"

Rest and leisure are part of any stage of life, but they are not life's purpose, fulfillment, or sole activity. Retirement is a time of transition that may begin with a euphoric honeymoon phase, during which the retiree gets involved with many things that were ruled out by full-time employment. During the second or third years of retirement, a degree of emotional letdown occurs, and seniors experience a crisis. If they are not involved in meaningful activities, their self-esteem and self-worth are shattered and depression ensues. For others, the life transition is a springboard to a new stage of life. The all-American saying "you are what you do; if you do nothing—you are nothing" expresses the deep-rooted work ethic that only through work or volunteering can life be fulfilled.

For many, the new stage starts with questions: What can I do? Where do I belong? What is my purpose? In order to make decisions about a new orientation in life, one has to look inward. Even though we are not always conscious of what life has in store for us, the potential design for our futures already exists in the spiritual cores of our real selves. We do not have conscious access to it, but occasionally the truth flushes out in a spiritual enlightenment and reveals to us our true purposes in life for which we were intended.

To start something new means to evolve along the spiritual continuum within ourselves toward goals and ideas that are an intrinsic part of our uniquenesses. What we want to accomplish has to be something that never was created by somebody else, something that evolved from our own individual experiences and potentials. If we imitate someone's ideas, we are not realizing the dormant talents stored in our true selves.

Some of the ancient books, such as Sanskrit literature, the Old and New Testaments, and others, refer to events where the true missions were revealed to people throughout history. Moses, faced with the burning bush, was enlightened about his mission to deliver his people out of the hands of Egyptians, and he accepted this titanic task. Abraham was tested by his God when he was asked to sacrifice his only son to prove the depth of his faith. Apostle Paul proclaimed the Lord Jesus as the personification of universal love and dedicated his life to spreading Christianity.

Millions of people have responded to the call and fulfilled their missions in life, but not all of them. When Jonas was called to save the city of Nineveh, a location reportedly filled with sinners, he decided to "flee…the presence of the Lord,"[4] took a boat, and refused to pursue his high assignment. According to the Old Testament, Jonas paid a high price for his rebellion: A huge fish swallowed him and he stayed inside the fish's belly for three days, symbolizing separation from life and God. Jonas then realized his mistake, repented, and was liberated from the unbearable isolation and guilt for failing the people of Nineveh.

The force of creativity reveals to us our talents and purposes in life, a realization that will make us fulfilled and abounding with vigor and energy. If we decline the "mission," our fates may be no better than the one of Jonas. If Christopher Columbus, Dr. Albert Schweitzer, or George Washington had refused their callings, the world would be immensely impoverished and changed by it. If all people on this planet refused to fulfill their purposes, the world would self-destruct. If the negativity of humankind would become greater than its capacity for love, compassion, hope, kindness, and faith, the energy field would regress to a destructive level.

Dr. David R. Hawkins, known for his research in the field of energy, stated that one godly person, such as Buddha or Jesus Christ, vibrates positive energy to the field that will counterbalance the negative forces of 750,000 individuals who emanate low, negative energy.[5] What great potential humankind has to elevate the world to a higher level of humaneness and peace, if only we could grow to the task.

Best-selling author Dr. Wayne W. Dyer made a revealing statement in his book *Inspiration: Your Ultimate Calling:*

You are here in your physical body; there was a time when you were an embryo; before that a seed, and before that formless energy. That formless energy contained intention that brought you from nowhere to now here. At the highest level of awareness, intention started you on a path toward your destiny.[6]

This inspiring statement by Dyer is a reminder of the miraculous moment of your conception, when the fertilized ovum was so small that it could not be perceived by the naked eye.[7] It weighed only 0.0015 milligrams, yet, it contained all your characteristics, including temperament, basic intelligence, skin, eye, and hair color, predisposition to physical conditions, as well as your unique talents and potential.

While the ovum you once were has multiplied 50 billion times to your current body size, other parts of your potential remain a mystery. The "Freudian" barrier between the conscious and unconscious parts of the psyche cannot be penetrated by logic or willpower.

Even though a basic potential was given to us in the form of genetic endowment at birth, our futures are not predetermined by it. We are in a continuous process of deliberate choice making during our lives. Our genetic equipment serves as a base from which to operate, but the spiritual connection to creativity is always present, even if we are not aware of it.

While we cannot predict our futures, we need to have a vision of life that is worth living. Campbell wrote that we have to follow our bliss. If we dedicate life only to materialistic pursuits, to the exclusion of our talents, life will gravitate toward crises and will be incomplete. The history of humanity is filled with examples of men and women who gave up life for "lucre," like Dr. Faust, and lost it. Others who did what they loved succeeded in a great way.

Charles Darwin studied medicine upon the insistence of his father who was also a physician. However, Darwin was not happy because his interests attracted him to natural sciences. After enduring two years of medical college, he quit, to the great disappointment of his father, and became a naturalist. Darwin's decision led not only to the personal fulfillment of his life, but also to his theories about the evolution of species, which became one of the leading contributions to the origins of humankind.[8]

Those who love what they do cannot stop doing what they love because it is their intended purposes. It brings them ongoing fulfillment and joy. Those who are still searching for their purposes in later years need to be open to all possibilities and look for inspiration that will lead them through creativity to unexpected discoveries of their potentials.

▪ ▪ ▪

What is creativity? What is its source? Why is it of special significance to seniors?

"Creativity is more important than knowledge," stated Albert Einstein. "Knowledge is limited, while creativity encircles the world."[9] To every stimulus, creative energy responds in a new way that is not based on old habits or patterns, but is generated and stimulated from a quantum source. Einstein once asked the poet Saint-John Perse how the idea of a poem came to him. The poet spoke about intuition and inspiration and Einstein responded, "It is the same for a man of science. It is a sudden illumination, almost a rapture. Later intelligent analyses and experiments confirm or invalidate the intuition."[10]

Creativity is one of the most powerful phenomena experienced by humankind. It can transform thoughts and actions and elevate them to a higher level of reality where inspiration enlightens new possibilities far beyond any expectations. Without the enigmatic power of creativity, we would not have Shakespeare, Mozart, and Goethe, light bulbs, television, or interplanetary rockets.

In the best seller *Inspiration: Your Ultimate Calling,* Dyer highlights a statement by Hindu philosopher Patañjali: "When you are inspired, dormant forces, facilities, and talents become alive, and you discover yourself to be a greater person by far than you ever dreamed yourself to be."[11]

If we know that creativity can elevate us to a higher level of being, why are we not seeking it with greater perseverance?

Modern people are so engaged in succeeding and achieving goals of material value that they forget the importance of their inner qualities. Life becomes materialistic and practical, and we are responding to never-ending demands and stimuli by habits, never having enough time to look inward where creativity begins. Because we are programmed by society to look for answers outside rather than within us, we lose touch with spiritual life.

Campbell confirms the alienation of modern people from their inner cores: "We are so engaged in doing things to achieve purpose of outer value that we forgot that the inner value, the rapture associated with being alive, is what it is all about."[12]

Moreover, new ideas upset people's fixed habits because they call them to respond in new ways to emerging circumstances. The possibility of change, even if it is toward something better, is disturbing because it requires risk and faith in oneself.

Some seniors do not believe that they can learn novel things. As we know, we are defined by what we believe. The only way we could fail is if we doubt that we will succeed. Those who do not believe in themselves project their doubts and lack of faith on their environments, which, in return, convey to them their own skepticism.

Creativity is of extraordinary importance for seniors because through its practice, they can increase energy and productivity at a time of diminishing physical options. Since the creative process is consistent with wisdom, it is a most welcome asset in later years when intellectual velocity may show some slowdown. Creativity regenerates our capacity for new achievements in unexpected ways. George B. Shaw, Leo Tolstoy, Pablo Picasso, or Chancellor Konrad Adenauer were actively creative into the ninth decade of life. It is well known that Picasso reinvented himself professionally from cubism to surrealism, futurism, pottery, drawing, and printmaking. Creative living is a vehicle for becoming alive and is rejuvenated by new ideas stemming from infinite sources.

Particle physics demonstrates that our bodies are separate entities to our senses only. In reality, we are part of vibrant energy waves of the universe, albeit in a different density and form. There is no activity in our cells that is not noticed by the field. Our bodies exist as creative potential inspired by the intelligence of the universe that physicists call the quantum field and theologians name God. When the universe talks to us, do we hear? When new possibilities emerge in our lives, do we see?

Chantal was an attractive, ambitious young woman determined to become a singer. She diligently worked toward her goal, perfecting her voice, using the influence of her father, a TV producer, for appearances, not missing any opportunity for a performance and publicity. Yet, after 10 years of life totally dedicated to her career, her goal to become a popular singer was not realized. She married a promising composer hoping that together they could become a popular duo. Her perseverance ended when her husband died in a car accident. Grieving and shattered, Chantal realized the emptiness of past years and the futility of her goal to be famous. She quit singing and, in financial distress, accepted an office job at an orphanage. There, her true potential became apparent: Her natural compassion and organizational talents were soon recognized by the administration. She participated in the rebuilding of this underfunded organization and helped to restore it through successful fundraising to become a secure home for abandoned children. Finally, she not only found the fulfillment that for many years of her past life was missing, Chantal realized that her misguided ambition for glory made her believe that she had artistic talent while she was unable to see her potential of much greater value.

Sciences can explain events rationally, but there is a point when they cannot unravel the incidents in our lives that occur without an apparent cause. When creative energy from the quantum field enlightens us with awareness of possibilities for full realization of our potential, can we follow?

Maslow developed the road map for the creative process of life. It was intended for everyone, regardless of age, culture, or health. He called it self-actualization. His system of thinking and doing encouraged all people to pursue their potentials toward greater humaneness. Other professionals followed his lead and enriched his seminal work by additional ideas. The following points are a summary of the salient guideposts that may enlighten the road less traveled by the experiences and insights of those who traveled the road before us.

- You are born for a purpose, and your purpose is the actualization of your potential.
- Creative living is a highway for the actualization of your potential.
- Your beliefs influence every cell in your body. Positive thoughts can change your biology and elevate you beyond entropy.
- Be inspired by your real self, by inspiring people, nature, arts, and spiritual literature.

- To resist your purpose in life may result in a feeling of disconnectedness and incompleteness.
- Join people with higher levels of energy. Avoid those who pollute your life.
- When in crisis, focus on love in your real self that is a source of support. Seek the support and love of others; it exists if you believe in it.
- Practice tolerance, kindness, compassion, and forgiveness. Avoid criticism, anger, selfishness, and revenge. As you give, it will be given to you.
- If you compete, compete with yourself: Be better today than you were yesterday. If you make a mistake, do not criticize yourself; continue to improve with persistence.
- Your creative energy will be amplified if you return it to the world through your work.

Anyone who has ever tried to call creativity into action knows that it does not respond to willpower, ego goals, or logic. If we believe in the existence of creativity, seek it as a lifelong resource, respect it as nature's precious gift, and use it with love for a purpose that counts, it will spontaneously appear when we need it most.

Grandma Moses was a farmer's wife who had to wait 76 years before she could do what she always liked: paint. Her wish came true only when she was no longer able to work on the farm. Her vision of rural life turned ordinary things into extraordinary dimensions. Were her reputation and fantastic earnings out of proportion with her talent? The material benefits would not have happened if it had not been for her determination to continue her creative work regardless of age, rural status, social expectations, and values. She self-actualized throughout her life.

The concept of creativeness and the concept of the healthy, self-actualizing, fully "human person seems to be...the same thing," states Maslow.[13] He further states,

Self-actualizing people are, without one single exception, involved in a cause, in something outside of them. They are devoted to working at something which is very precious to them, some call it vocation in the old sense. They are working at something which fate has called them to do and which they love, so that the work-joy dichotomy disappears. One devotes life to the law, another to the beauty or truth.[14]

One of those who found his fulfillment in the practice of psychiatry was Carl Jung. "My life is a story of the self-realization of the unconscious," he admitted.[15]

When our work is done, is there a difference between a peak experience emanating from the contemplation of an art work that we created, or from gazing at a field of golden wheat that we seeded and that is growing in the sun under the blue skies?

Einstein referred to the peak experience as the "cosmic religious feelings," which relates to a sublime state beyond dogma or sciences that connects us to the universal Source as a unifying power of humanity.[16]

What was the most creative moment of your life? Have you experienced an unforgettable moment of spiritual elation that transcended the limitations of here and now?

Maslow writes that it is not easy to talk about transcendental feelings—they are kept private—because it is not "scientific" to discuss them in public. In his opinion there is always a trigger that starts an experience that sort of gravitates toward a spiritual climax. The most common peak experiences are achieved through personal intimate relationships, or through accomplishment of a creative endeavor that was pursued with passion and dedication.[17] For an astrophysicist to detect a new galaxy or to discover some of the universe's secrets may lead to a moment of transcendent ecstasy, as well as for a poet's completion of an inspiring work that will ignite feelings of beauty in others. Sublime moments are reported by some actors and opera singers who gave themselves entirely to the performance or by runners who achieved an extraordinary physical record that superseded their expectations. A climber who reached the top of a mountain and sees the world under his feet or an astronomer who views our planet for the first time both experience peak moments of unforgettable intensity. Mother Teresa reported peak moments every day by helping the poorest of poor in Calcutta: In every one of them, she saw the Lord Jesus.

Maslow also refers to childbearing as a mystical experience—an illumination, a revelation, an insight, leading to a peak experience that results in, what he called, "the cognition of being." Maslow elaborated that this "cognition of being" is a "technology of happiness, of pure excellence, pure truth, pure goodness." Peak experiences are a unique way to help people, who feel empty, to discover what emotions are like. They are signals from inside that yell at you: "By gosh, this is good, don't even doubt it," adds Maslow.[18]

The path toward self-actualization through the creative process of life and the discovery of self is open to people of all ages who want to walk the road less traveled.

Your creativity is waiting to be called into action.

7 ■ ■ ■

Eating to Live Stronger, Live Longer

NANCY M. RYAN, M.S., R.D., C.D.E.

> Above all—try something.
>
> —Franklin Delano Roosevelt

Jack, an 80-year-"young" patient of mine, starts his day with a brisk walk. He chooses his foods wisely to keep his diabetes and cholesterol under control. He reviews his medications and supplements with his doctor at his regularly scheduled visits. Jack's only complaint is that there are not enough hours in the day to accomplish all of the tasks on his formidable "to do" list.

In contrast, Joe is 51 years "old" and struggles to make it through his day. He never seems to have time to exercise and eats on the run. As his waist size has increased, his blood pressure and blood cholesterol have also. His doctor recently told him that his blood glucose (sugar) is creeping up. Joe says he wants to take better care of himself, but is feeling overwhelmed.

> It's not the years in your life but the life in your years that counts.
>
> —Adlai Stevenson

When entering this new phase in our lives, it is important to remember that our present health reflects a complex history of genetics and lifestyle choices. While we cannot change our genes, the new field of nutragenomics may reveal the impact of foods on "gene expression," or turning on beneficial genes and turning off genes that can lead to deleterious changes in our bodies.

There is a plethora of research on the impact of lifestyle, including diet and physical activity, on one's health. What is not always clear in the reports we read and see in the public media is the strength of the research and recommendations that come forth from the studies. For health-care consumers, it can be very challenging to separate well-supported recommendations from those that are intriguing and provocative, but not yet corroborated. Major health associations, such as the American Diabetes Association, the American Heart Association, and the American Cancer Society, have addressed this issue within their communities of experts and health practitioners, assigning a level of evidence to general recommendations that reflects the strength of the supporting research. In summarizing nutrition recommendations for our later years, we will attempt to indicate strength of the recommendations in a fashion similar to this. I encourage the reader to examine all nutrition claims and recommendations with a critical eye.

The science of nutrition is an active area of study. Dietary recommendations may change over time as more and stronger evidence becomes available. While at times it appears that recommendations change dramatically from week to week, the reality is that the basic tenets of eating will remain: Choose fruits, vegetables, whole grains, low fat or nonfat dairy products, lean protein, and "heart-healthy" fats. This advice is not glamorous or showy, but it is well corroborated by solid research.

As a traveler on this journey of healthful aging, consider these caveats:

- "Natural" does not equal "safe." There have been numerous documented cases of injury and death from nutrition products touted as natural.[1] Many of the medications used today were derived from plants. Herbal products may have compounds with strong medicinal effects, but not the necessary quality control of medications.
- "More" does not equal "better." Even something as seemingly innocuous as vitamin C can cause health problems when taken in excess.[2]
- Always review with your physician(s) any dietary supplements and herbal products you take. Do this at each visit with your doctor. It is very common for many of us to be taking multiple medications. There may be

interactions between medications and supplements or herbals that can interfere with the way our medicines work, either decreasing the effect or magnifying the effect.[3]

■ FEEDING THE MASTER CONTROLS OF THE BODY

The master controls of the body, the immune, nervous, and endocrine systems, work in unique and coordinated ways to keep these complex machines we call our bodies functioning at maximum performance levels. Our food choices interact with these master controls in varied ways to keep us energized and engaged with our world. Conditions associated with increasing age, but not caused by it, such as heart disease, arthritis, or diabetes, can influence our abilities to be full, active participants in a vibrant life. Lifestyle choices, such as eating a healthy diet, can help us control and sometimes avoid these chronic ills.

Below, I have tried to summarize a number of these interactions in describing how food choices can sustain and improve health. Be aware that this is not a comprehensive presentation of all the research and recommendations in these areas. Rather, it is a snapshot of considerations and possibilities. It may be a starting point for some who are struggling to begin committing to better eating. For others, it may be corroboration that they are on the right track and, perhaps, can apply additional "fine-tuning" to their diets. The challenge is to begin.

■ ENERGY: FUELING OUR HEALTH

Are you regularly choosing to eat "high-octane" foods? I asked Jack this question and, not surprisingly, he makes sure that each day he includes plenty of fruits, vegetables, whole grains, and lean protein-rich foods in his meals and snacks. Joe, on the other hand, relies on foods that are convenient and fast, often skips meals and overeats later in the day, and snacks on salty, fatty chips and fries. It is not surprising, then, that Joe says he is tired all day long and has little interest in pursuing leisure activities including exercise, while Jack is on the go and enjoying his life.

High-octane foods are more appropriately called nutrient-dense foods. These are foods that provide not only needed calories to fuel those biological "machines" in each of our body's cells, but they are rich sources of vitamins, minerals, fiber, and phytochemicals that maintain each cell in top working order. Each decade after our 20s, our calorie or energy needs slowly and gradually decline, but not our need for the nutrients for health, some of which actually increase.[4] It takes organization and planning to ensure that most of our food choices are nutrient dense with calories sufficient to maintain a healthy weight.

Approach each day as an opportunity to eat well. Organization and planning begins before the trip to the market. Build your shopping list from the nutrient-dense foods as suggested below. Each day, consider your schedule and plans. Make a strategy for building in meals and snacks: What will I eat, when will I eat, where will I eat? Without a game plan, achieving our objective of vigor and health is nearly impossible.

Table 7.1   Nutrient-Dense Foods and Daily Servings*

Food	Portion	Servings per Day*
Nonfat or low-fat dairy	1 cup skim or 1 percent milk, 1 cup yogurt, or 1½ ounces low-fat cheese	3
Vegetables	½ cup cooked, nonstarchy vegetables; ½ cup vegetable or tomato juice (preferably lower sodium), or 1 cup raw vegetables/salad	4–5
Fruit	1 small piece of fresh fruit, 1 cup melon, ¾ cup berries, or 1 small banana	4–5
Grains	1 slice whole grain bread, ½–1 cup high-fiber cereal, ⅓ cup pasta, rice, or noodles, 1 medium potato, or 1 small yam	6–8
Protein-rich foods	Poultry, fish, lean red meat, beans, lentils, dried peas, tofu, soy-based "burgers," eggs, peanut butter, or low-fat cheese	6 ounces
Heart-healthy fat	Olive oil, canola oil, nuts, seeds, peanut butter, or avocado	1–2 tablespoons

* General recommendations; number of servings may vary based upon calorie needs.
Source: Adapted from Dietary Guidelines for Americans 2005; www.health.gov/dietaryguidelines and DASH Eating Plan 2006; www.nhlbi.nih.gov.

Regular refueling of our bodies with nutrient-dense foods is a critical requirement for sustaining energy throughout the day. Skipping or postponing meals, as is Joe's habit, deprives the body of the fuel or calories it needs for the work of the day, as well as the nutrients that help to drive that work. While there is no hard and fast rule regarding meal times, a good practice is to limit the time between eating, whether meals or snacks, to no more than 4 to 5 hours.

Besides food consumption, hydration affects one's energy level during the day. Inadequate fluid intake can lead to fatigue and is sometimes misinterpreted as hunger, leading to overeating. Generally, 6 to 8 eight-ounce servings of fluid each day meet the needs of most people. The best fluid is water. Other reasonable fluids include milk, fruit juice, caffeine-free tea and coffee, and seltzer. Again, planning can be the key to meeting our fluid needs. Keep a pitcher of water in the refrigerator and work on finishing it each day. Take bottled water with you if you will be away from home during the day.

Energy robbers need to be considered. These include certain medical conditions, inadequate or poor sleep, alcohol, tobacco, and lack of physical activity. Medical conditions, such as a low-functioning thyroid or undiagnosed or poorly controlled diabetes, can cause significant fatigue and must be discussed with your doctor. Most of us need seven to nine hours of restorative sleep each night. Alcohol and tobacco can interfere with restorative sleep. Regular physical activity increases muscle strength and tone, oxygen and nutrient delivery to all organ systems, and assists in getting a good night's sleep.

■ FEEDING THE SKIN WE ARE IN

Who greets you in the morning when you look in the mirror? Do you see a bright-eyed, glowing reflection of yourself? Or, do you see a pale, sallow, lackluster stranger? What you see is what the world sees. This visible representation we project to the world defines how the world categorizes us.

Skin is the largest organ in our bodies, responsible for protecting our internal organs, providing a barrier to repel infections, and controlling internal temperature. Normal processes of metabolism produce by-products called reactive oxygen species (ROS) that have been implicated in the aging process. The skin is constantly exposed to ROS

Table 7.2   Dietary Components' Affects on Skin

Skin-Protective Foods and Nutrients	Foods and Nutrients Associated with Greater Skin Wrinkling
Vegetables (especially green leafy vegetables, eggplant, asparagus, celery, onion, and garlic)	Red meat
Olive oil, olives, and monounsaturated fats	Full-fat dairy products (such as whole milk, butter, and ice cream)
Legumes (especially broad and lima beans)	Sweets[‡]
Skim milk	Margarine
Fermented milk products (yogurt and cheese)	Vitamin C[*]
Nuts	
Fruit (such as cherries, grapes, melon, prunes, apples, and pears)	
Multigrain bread	
Jam	
Tea	
Water	
Fish (although the evidence was weaker than for the above foods)	
Nutrients: iron, zinc, calcium, phosphorus, magnesium, retinol (vitamin A), and vitamin C[*,†]	

[*] Vitamin C acts as an antioxidant at recommended daily intake levels. At high levels, vitamin C can act as a pro-oxidant, which the study authors theorized when the statistical analysis associated high vitamin C intakes in study participants with increased markers of skin aging. [†] Of note, these nutrients were from the foods consumed in the studies, not added as dietary supplements. [‡] By raising blood glucose/sugar, proteins and other components of the skin's cells undergo a process called glycosylation, which has been implicated in enhanced skin aging.

Source: Martalena br Purba, et al., "Skin Wrinkling: Can Food Make a Difference?" *Journal of the American College of Nutrition* 20, no. 1 (2001): 71–80.

through sun exposure and the blood flow to the skin with delivery of nutrients, oxygen, as well as ROS. It is believed that antioxidants from one's diet combat the damaging effects of ROS and thus the appearance of the skin.

Can our diet and food choices affect skin health and aging? An international study conducted by researchers in Australia, Greece, and Sweden attempted to determine if the food choices we make can affect skin wrinkling and aging changes.[5] They found there were foods and nutrients that were associated with less skin wrinkling in their older adult subjects, as well as foods associated with greater degrees of skin wrinkling.

Vitamin A and beta-carotene (which the body converts to vitamin A) support and heal the epithelial cells of the skin. Nonfat dairy foods, egg yolks, liver, and fatty fish are some rich sources of vitamin A. Foods rich in beta-carotene include orange and red fruits and vegetables, such as cantaloupe, apricots, peaches, pink grapefruit, tomatoes, yams, carrots, pumpkin, and winter squash. Dark green vegetables, such as spinach, greens, broccoli, and asparagus, are also good sources of beta-carotene. There is some limited evidence that beta-carotene may also help protect the skin against sun damage, perhaps enhancing the protective effect of sunscreens.[6]

Vitamin C is known to be essential for collagen production in the body. Collagen, a protein that supports skin structure, becomes damaged over time with exposure to the sun. In its role as an antioxidant, vitamin C exerts a protective effect against cellular damage by free radicals, highly reactive and destructive compounds naturally produced as a part of normal metabolism. Vitamin C rich foods include citrus fruit (i.e., oranges, grapefruit, and tangerines), strawberries, cantaloupe, cruciferous vegetables (i.e., cabbage, Brussels sprouts, and broccoli), greens, and tomatoes. Of note, an excess intake of vitamin C may act as a pro-oxidant and thus may promote skin aging.[7]

The antioxidant properties of vitamin E are recognized. Vitamin E may also protect tissues, including skin cells, by decreasing the production of collagenase, a protein enzyme that breaks down the support tissue collagen, and increasing the production of connective tissue growth factor.[8] Foods rich in vitamin E include vegetable oils, nuts, wheat germ, and whole grain breads and cereals.

The impact of genistein, a phytoestrogen derived from soybeans, on postmenopausal symptom reduction, bone health, and cardiovascular disease has been examined for many years. More recently, the role of genistein in skin protection from aging related to sun exposure and reduced risk of skin cancer has become a focus of research. In animal and human studies, genistein has reduced the inflammation from exposure to

Table 7.3   Isoflavone Content of Soy-Based Foods

Food	Approximate Portion	Milligrams of Isoflavones
Edamame	½ cup	20
Soy burgers	3 ounces	8–9
Miso	½ cup	40
Natto	½ cup	60
Soybeans, raw	½ cup	60–145
Soy cheese	3 ounces	6–30
Soy flour	½ cup	130–210
Soy milk	1 cup	20
Tempeh	½ cup	40–50
Tofu	½ cup	20–30

Source: U.S. Department of Agriculture, Agricultural Research Service. 2007. USDA–Iowa State University Database on the Isoflavone Content of Foods, Release 1.4—2007. Nutrient Data Laboratory Web site: http://www.ars.usda.gov/nutrientdata.

ultraviolet radiation.[9] Genistein is the major isoflavone in soy. Above is a list of soy-based foods and their approximate isoflavone content.[10]

Just as hydration helps maintain one's energy level, it is also vital to good skin health. The general recommendation of 6 to 8 eight-ounce servings of fluid, preferably water, helps maintain skin suppleness.

■ SYSTEMIC INFLAMMATION

Systemic inflammation is a term scientists use to describe a complex interaction between hormones and tissues in the body that increase the risk of chronic illness, such as heart disease, high blood pressure, and type 2 diabetes. With an increase in the amount of fat one carries deep within the abdomen (called visceral fat), there is a change in the production of certain hormones, such as adiponectin and resistin, that leads to a cascade of events that make our blood vessels less pliable and smooth, causing blood pressure to rise and cholesterol to deposit and form plaques. Insulin becomes less effective in regulating blood glucose or sugar, setting the stage for diabetes.

Doctors test for systemic inflammation by looking at a marker in the blood called cardiac or high sensitivity c-reactive protein (cCRP or hsCRP). If this nonspecific marker is elevated, we may be advised to take aspirin.

Additional strategies to address systemic inflammation include the following:

- maintaining a healthy weight,
- eating fatty fish two or more times per week, and
- consuming foods rich in anti-inflammatory phytonutrients.

Fatty or oily fish, such as salmon, tuna, and sardines, are rich in omega-3 fats, particularly DHA (docosahexaenoic acid) and EPA (eicosapentaenoic acid). These omega-3 fats have been found to reduce the body's production of compounds implicated in systemic inflammation.[11] The recommended target for DHA + EPA is about 400–500 mg (milligrams) per day, which can be met by eating about 8 ounces of oily fish over the course of a week. For nonfish eaters, supplementation with omega-3 fats is a reasonable alternative. Look for the DHA and EPA content on the Nutrition Information portion of the supplement label to determine the amount of these omega-3 fats in the supplement. For vegetarians, an algeal-based supplement may be more acceptable. CAVEAT: Always review with your doctor the appropriateness of a supplement for you before starting to take it. While omega-3 or fish oil supplements have not been shown to be harmful in general, there may be reasons why a specific individual should not take them.

Phytonutrient is the term given to components in foods that are not vitamins or minerals, but appear to have significant health benefits. A number of phytonutrients, such as resveratrol, have been found to tamp down the body's inflammatory response. Foods rich in resveratrol include red grapes, berries, and peanuts. Other phytonutrients believed to have anti-inflammatory effects in the body include carotenoids (in yellow, orange, and dark green vegetables and fruit), catechins (in green tea and cocoa), and theaflavins (in black tea), to name just a few. In general, fruits, vegetables, and whole grains are rich sources of phytonutrients.

▪ EATING SMART FOR YOUR HEART

Heart disease is a leading cause of death and disability in the United States. Keeping our hearts and circulatory systems healthy is a lifelong effort. Even if we have heart or vascular disease, it is never too late to eat smart for our hearts. Strategies for a heart-healthy lifestyle include the following:

- maintaining a healthy weight;
- choosing the fats in our diet wisely: monounsaturated fat (MUFA), poly-unsaturated fat (PUFA), and saturated fat (SFA) balance;
- eating foods rich in soluble fiber and phytosterols; and
- remaining physically active.

The traditional blood lipid profile, that is, the blood test measuring the amount of total cholesterol, LDL (low-density liprotein), HDL (high-density lipoprotein), and triglycerides, helps our doctors assess our risks of developing heart and vascular disease. More recently, tests looking at the size and density of LDL and HDL particles as well as other fats in our blood, such as VLDL (very low-density lipoprotein), IDL (intermediate-density lipoprotein), and LP(a) ("ugly" cholesterol), have become available. These tests can flesh out the risk portraits our doctors view. The LDL particle that is small and dense appears to be more athero-genic, i.e., causing plaque deposition and buildup in artery walls. LDL that is "light and buoyant," while not risk-free, appears to be less athero-genic. Likewise, large HDL appears to be more protective against plaque buildup, while small, dense HDL appears to be less protective.

The balance of fats in our diets affects the markers of heart disease risk that our doctors monitor with us. LDL cholesterol, associated with plaque buildup in our arteries, and HDL cholesterol, associated with reduced risk of plaque buildup, can be altered based upon the foods we eat. Altering this balance is as easy as changing our dietary fat profiles:[12]

Omega-3 Fats and Heart Disease

There is good evidence that omega-3 fats are heart healthy. In the Nurses Health Study, those women with the highest consumption of fish had a decreased risk of coronary heart disease (CHD).[13] In the Physician's Health Study, the risk of sudden cardiac death was lower for those individuals with the highest fish intake.[14] It has been estimated that for each 20 gram per day increase in fish (which is ⅔ of an ounce of fish), the risk of death from CHD is lowered by about 7 percent.

Table 7.4   Dietary Fat Recommendations

Fat	Food Sources	Recommendation
MUFA	Olive oil, canola oil, peanut oil, nuts, seeds, and peanut butter (preferably natural)	Best choices
PUFA	Corn, safflower, sunflower, cottonseed oils, margarines, and mayonnaise	Use sparingly. Too much PUFA vs MUFA can cause HDL cholesterol to drop.
SFA	Butter, bacon, fatback, cream cheese, sour cream, and cream; also, the fat in fatty cuts of meat (fats that tend to be solid at room temperature)	Limit or avoid. These fats raise LDL cholesterol levels.
Trans fats	Listed as hydrogenated fat on food labels	Limit or avoid. These fats raise LDL cholesterol levels.
Omega-3 fats	Oily fish	Eat at least 2 servings per week of oily fish, such as salmon, tuna, sardines.

Source: Third Report of the National Cholesterol Education Program (NCEP) Expert Panel on Detection, Evaluation, and Treatment of High Blood Cholesterol in Adults (Adult Treatment Panel III). National Institutes of Health Publication No. 02-5215, September 2002.

In 2002, the American Heart Association first put forth recommendations for fish consumption to increase omega-3 fat intake. For individuals without CHD, eating fatty fish at least two times per week was recommended. This would provide on average of about 400–500 mg per day of omega-3 fats from about 8 ounces of fish over the course of a week. For individuals with heart disease, an intake of about 1,000 mg per day of EPA + DHA was recommended. For those individuals with high triglyceride levels in their blood, an intake of 2,000–3,000 mg per day of EPA + DHA was recommended. At these higher levels of intake, taking a dietary supplement becomes a consideration.[15,16]

The number of foods on the market with added omega-3 fats has increased in response to individuals looking for strategies to increase these fats in their diets. It is important to read food labels carefully to determine the amount and type of omega-3 fat that is in the food item. CAVEAT: At this time, it appears that the most potent omega-3 fats are the marine or fish fats: EPA and DHA. Alpha-linolenic acid (ALA) is also an omega-3 fat, rich sources of which include flax seed, flax seed oil, soybean oil, and canola oil. The impact of ALA on health is not fully understood. Only a very small amount of ALA that we eat is converted into EPA and DHA. Foods that have been supplemented with omega-3 fats may have ALA as opposed to EPA or DHA added.

Phytosterols

Phytosterols are naturally occurring compounds that are found in the membranes of plant foods. Two of these, sterols and stanols, are known to block the absorption of cholesterol from the intestinal tract. Foods that contain these compounds include fruits, vegetables, nuts and seeds, legumes (such as dried beans, peas, and lentils), grains, and vegetable oils. Studies exploring the impact of sterols and stanols have used much larger doses than foods can naturally provide. So, nutraceuticals, that is, foods with medicinal qualities, have been developed, such as butterlike spreads that are rich sources of these compounds. It has been demonstrated that including 2 to 3 grams of sterols or stanols each day can reduce LDL cholesterol in the blood by 6 to 15 percent.[17]

■ TAKING THE PRESSURE OFF: HYPERTENSION

For every three people you know, it is likely that one will have hypertension or high blood pressure. With increasing age, our risk of high blood pressure increases. The impact of high blood pressure on one's health includes a higher risk of stroke, heart attack, and kidney failure. If diabetes is present, high blood pressure also damages the delicate blood vessels in the eyes resulting in retinopathy, which can progress to blindness.[18,19]

These grim realities need to be recognized as uncontrolled hypertension is a leading cause of death and disability.

Yet, there are lifestyle interventions that we can put into place to control blood pressure. In the 1990s two seminal studies looked at the impact of the foods we eat on blood pressure. These two studies were part of the Dietary Approaches to Stop Hypertension (DASH) Trial.[20] The DASH Trials demonstrated a significant decrease in blood pressure when the study participants ate a diet rich in

Table 7.5   What Is Hypertension?

Blood Pressure Category	Systolic (upper number)	Diastolic (lower number)
Normal	Less than 120	Less than 80
"Prehypertension"	120–139	80–89
Hypertension		
Stage 1	140–159	90–99
Stage 2	Greater than 160	Greater than 100

Source: The Seventh Report of the Joint National Committee on Prevention, Detection, Evaluation, and Treatment of High Blood Pressure (JNC 7). NIH Publication No. 04-5230, August 2004.

- fruits and vegetables (about 8–10 servings per day),
- whole grains (about 8 servings per day),
- low-fat or fat-free dairy (3 servings per day),
- poultry, fish, and lean red meat (about 6 ounces per day),
- nuts and seeds (4–5 small servings per week),
- limited additional fat (heart-healthy) and sweets, and
- sodium (salt) intake of about 2,300 mg per day (in the second DASH trial).

After two weeks on the DASH diet, blood pressure was lowered to a degree similar to that which would be expected with a first-line antihypertension medication. The blood pressure lowering effect was maintained for the duration of the study.

This work underscores the power of the foods we eat on our health. Following the DASH recommendations may not preclude the need for medication to control blood pressure for some, but it may enhance the effectiveness of medications in controlling blood pressure.

▪ DIABETES

Over 21 million people in the United States have diabetes. One in three affected individuals does not even know he or she has this serious disorder. It has been estimated that at least 54 million additional people are in the pipeline, on their way to developing diabetes. These startling statistics are reflected in health-care costs where one out of every seven health care dollars spent is on diabetes.[21]

Table 7.6   Risk Factors for Type 2 Diabetes

Increasing age
Family history
Ethnicity: Native Americans, African Americans, Latinos/Hispanics, and Asian/Pacific Islanders
Sedentary lifestyle
Increased abdominal or visceral fat stores
History of gestational diabetes or giving birth to a baby weighing 9 or more pounds
History of polycystic ovary syndrome

Source: American Diabetes Association, "Standards of Medical Care in Diabetes—2008," *Diabetes Care* 31, no. 1 (2008): S12–S54.

The two major classifications of diabetes, type 1 (formerly known as insulin dependent or juvenile diabetes) and type 2 (formerly known as noninsulin dependent or adult onset) share some common characteristics, such as elevated blood glucose (sugar), but are actually two very different disorders. For our discussion, we will concentrate on type 2 diabetes.

Type 2 diabetes occurs most frequently in adults, but, with the growing obesity epidemic, children and adolescents are developing it. Diagnosis is made when blood glucose (sugar) exceeds a certain level (i.e., greater than 126 mg/dl [milligrams per deciliter] when fasting on at least two different occasions or greater than 200 mg/dl at any time of the day). Be mindful that elevated blood glucose is a late marker of diabetes. By the time the diagnostic criteria are met, there have been deleterious changes in the body occurring over the past 7 to 10 years. So, when newly diagnosed patients tell me they were recently told they have diabetes, I remind them that the diagnosis is new; trouble had been brewing well before that point.

More recently, type 2 diabetes has been described as a "vasculopathy," or a disease affecting the blood vessels of the body before blood glucose even begins to rise. As with heart disease, systemic inflammation appears to play a key role in the development of type 2 diabetes.

The purpose in emphasizing this point is that potential chronic complications may already have developed, and diabetes needs to be intensively managed at this point. Also, for those individuals at high risk of developing type 2 diabetes, that is, those in the pipeline with "prediabetes" (better described as impaired fasting glucose or impaired glucose tolerance), there is very good evidence that lifestyle intervention can significantly reduce the chances of going on to develop type 2 diabetes. The good news is that the lifestyle recommendations for type 2 diabetes and prediabetes are the same: Choose healthy foods, reduce weight if appropriate, and be physically active.

The most effective dietary modifications are those that have been individually tailored by the individual with diabetes in collaboration with his or her registered dietitian. General recommendations for eating well for diabetes include the following:

- In general, the less processed a food is, the less impact it has on raising blood glucose.
- Limit portion sizes, but do not omit foods that contain carbohydrates, such as cereals, breads, fruits, and milk.
- Try to include a small amount of heart-healthy fat at meals and snacks. This can help temper the rise in blood glucose after eating. (See the section "Eating Smart for Your Heart.")
- Avoid foods concentrated in sugar, such as fruit juices, cakes, pies, cookies, sweetened sodas, and beverages.
- Incorporate the "Eating Smart for Your Heart" recommendations as elevated blood lipids are a common problem in type 2 diabetes.

Medical Nutrition Therapy (MNT) is a Medicare Part B covered benefit for individuals with a diagnosis of diabetes. Physician referral is required and the registered dietitian must be a Medicare provider. Three hours of MNT are covered the first year the benefit is used. Each year thereafter, two hours of MNT are covered.

▊ KEEPING THE TWINKLE IN OUR EYES

Macular degeneration is the most common cause of vision loss and blindness in adults in the United States as well as worldwide. By our mid-70s, one in four people has early signs of age-related macular degeneration (AMD). Of the estimated 8 million individuals with intermediate AMD, about 16 percent will go on to develop advanced AMD within five years. The cause(s) of AMD and, most importantly, ways to prevent or slow down its progression are actively being pursued by researchers.

A number of studies[22–26] have examined nutritional interventions to slow the progression of AMD. A diet high in fat, particularly animal-derived fat, has been implicated in contributing to the progression of AMD. Vegetable oils, as well, have been implicated, while fat from fish and nuts may reduce the risk of progression. Some researchers suggest that AMD shares many characteristics with heart disease. For example, increased risk of progression of AMD is associated with abdominal obesity. Vigorous exercise appears to decrease risk.

Results of the Age-Related Eye Disease Study (AREDS) and Rotterdam studies suggested that high intakes of antioxidant nutrients, such as vitamin C, vitamin E, beta-carotene, and zinc may reduce the risk of AMD and slow progression to more advanced stages. Of interest, the Rotterdam Study used foods rich in these nutrients (as opposed to supplements) and found a 35 percent lower risk of AMD in individuals consuming a diet providing vitamin C, vitamin E, beta-carotene, and zinc at levels above the recommended dietary allowance. The role of phytonutrients, such as zeaxanthin and lutein, and omega-3 fats (DHA and EPA) in preventing or delaying the progression of AMD is currently being investigated in the AREDS II study.

The total carbohydrate intake as a risk factor for AMD has been examined and did not appear to increase cases of AMD. However, the after-meal blood glucose spikes, as suggested by the Glycemic Index of the diet, did appear to increase the risk of developing AMD. While this very interesting finding needs to be corroborated by further study, incorporating recommendations for blood glucose control (see ''Diabetes'') could control for this possible risk.

While answers regarding prevention and slowing down the progression of AMD are sought, incorporating the following into our diets would seem prudent:

- Include vegetables and fruits every day.
- Include fish (particularly fatty fish) at least two times per week.
- Include nuts several times per week.
- Limit total fat intake, including that from red meat and oils.

If you find these recommendations to appear similar to those for managing heart health, blood pressure, diabetes, you are correct!

■ FEEDING THE BRAIN

Probably one of the most frightening aspects to aging is loss of cognitive function. Sure, many of us have trouble remembering where we put our sunglasses. Of greater concern is if we find those sunglasses in the freezer!

Eating to keep the brain and the nervous system healthy, in general, is the same as eating to keep the heart healthy. Maintaining one's blood lipids, blood pressure, and blood glucose at the targets set with one's doctor helps reduce the risk of transient ischemic attacks ("mini-strokes") and stroke.

In addition to decreasing the risk for stroke, dietary manipulation to slow the decline in brain or cognitive function has been examined. In the Nurses Health Study,[27] those study participants with the highest reported consumption of vegetables (particularly green, leafy vegetables and cruciferous vegetables, such as broccoli, cauliflower, cabbage, and kale), had the slowest rate of decrease in cognitive function. No relation was found between cognitive decline and fruit consumption.

There is also interesting evidence suggesting fish truly is brain food. The omega-3 fat, DHA, may protect the brain from changes leading to dementia and Alzheimer's disease. Examination of brains from individuals with dementia and Alzheimer's disease showed lower levels of DHA than the brains of those not exhibiting cognitive decline prior to death. Increased fish and DHA intake have been associated with slower cognitive decline. In one study, there was a 60 percent decrease in the risk of developing Alzheimer's disease when fish was eaten at least once a week. In studies of mice, supplementation with DHA prevented or delayed the onset of Alzheimer's disease.[28]

A phytochemical found in the spice turmeric, curcumin, has been shown to be a powerful anti-inflammatory and antioxidant. In mice studies, supplements of curcumin reduced the amount of amyloid plaque that formed in the brain. Amyloid plaques are one of the changes seen in the brain structure of individuals with Alzheimer's disease.[29]

Again, in mice studies of Alzheimer's disease, a low-calorie diet decreased the buildup of amyloid plaque in the brain.[30] It is too big a leap from mice to people, but these findings certainly are provocative.

The upshot regarding our diets and brain health would be the following:

- Choose the fats in our diet wisely: a MUFA, PUFA, and SFA balance.
- Maintain a healthy weight.
- Remain physically active.
- Include vegetables and fruits every day.
- Include fish (particularly fatty fish) at least two times per week.
- Include nuts several times per week.
- Limit total and saturated fat intake.

ARTHRITIS

Swollen, hot, and tender joints are characteristics of both osteoarthritis ("wear-and-tear" arthritis) and rheumatoid arthritis (arthritis caused by a malfunctioning of the body's own immune system). There have been many popular dietary remedies proposed over the years, many of which have yet to be proven. For instance, avoiding nightshade vegetables (that is, potato, green pepper, eggplant, and tomato) has not been shown to consistently improve the symptoms of arthritis. Eating butter to keep the joints "lubricated" is also a proposed but unfounded treatment for arthritis.

There is, however, some very provocative evidence that omega-3 fats (DHA and EPA) can moderate the inflammation seen in rheumatoid arthritis (RA). In studies in which omega-3 fat supplements were given as an average dose of about 3.5 grams per day, patients reported fewer tender and swollen joints, less morning stiffness, increased grip strength, and less use of anti-inflammatory medications. Some researchers have suggested that reducing the amount of omega-6 fats (i.e., vegetable oils) while increasing omega-3 fats can have an even greater impact on RA symptoms.[31]

Phytochemicals, such as catechins in green tea and carotenoids in orange and yellow fruits and vegetables, may reduce the risk of RA and osteoarthritis (OA), according to animal and limited human studies.

Maintaining a healthy weight is indirectly beneficial to joint health. Less pressure on affected joints reduces pain and swelling in OA.

While the efficacy of minerals and phytochemicals in the diet needs further study, the impact of omega-3 fish oils for RA is recognized. General guidelines include the following:

- Maintain a healthy weight.
- Include fish (particularly fatty fish) at least two times per week.

- Discuss with your primary doctor and/or rheumatologist the addition of omega-3 fish oil supplements to your treatment regimen.
- Include vegetables and fruits every day, particularly deep yellow and orange varieties.
- Drink green tea during the day.

■ INTESTINAL HEALTH

The intestinal tract is a hub of activity, beginning at the mouth and ending at the anus. In addition to its role in food digestion and nutrient absorption, it secretes hormones that help regulate appetite, advance digested food through the tract via peristalsis, and interacts with insulin to enable us to use the carbohydrates, proteins, and fats we consume. The intestine also is a protective barrier against noxious substances and a producer of compounds such as vitamin K via the healthy bacteria that reside primarily in the large intestine.

Supporting the healthy bacteria in the intestine reduces the risk of illness from pathogenic or illness-causing bacteria and other micro-organisms in the gut. Much research has been done, and is still ongoing, regarding the use of probiotics for a healthy intestine. "Probiotics" have been defined by the international body Food and Agricultural Organization:World Health Organization (FAO:WHO) Working Group as "live microorganisms which, when administered in adequate amounts, confer a health benefit on the host,"[32] i.e., you. Probiotics have been used for centuries in the form of cultured dairy products, such as yogurt and kefir, and fermented soy products, such as tempeh and miso.

There is evidence that certain strains of probiotics may help ulcerative colitis in individuals to remain in remission. They may also help prevent a relapse in individuals with Crohn's disease. Research into the impact of probiotics in irritable bowel syndrome, H. pylori infection, tooth decay and periodontal disease, vaginal infections, and skin infections is ongoing. There is preliminary evidence the certain strains of probiotics may reduce the recurrence of bladder cancer. Probiotics may also decrease the length of time of infection by Clostridium difficile, a bacteria that causes significant diarrhea.[33]

"Prebiotics" are compounds from foods that help support the healthy gut bacteria. These include such compounds as inulin, fructo-oligosaccharides, polydextrose, and polyols. Food sources of prebiotics include whole grains, bananas, garlic, onions, leeks, and honey, to name a few. Prebiotics have been shown to increase calcium and magnesium absorption in the intestine. They also may slow down or stop precancerous lesions in the intestine.

"Synbiotics" is the term used to describe foods or supplements that include both probiotics and prebiotics.

Foods to which probiotics are added have been introduced to the food market. While there is evidence that certain types of bacteria, such as Bifidobacteria and Lactobacilli, may confer health benefits, some researchers caution that one must consider the genus, the species, and the strain of the bacteria added to a food as they all do not act in the same fashion. Also, safety issues need to be addressed, particularly for individuals with compromised immune systems, which will include some elderly.

The impact of omega-3 fat on inflammatory bowel disease (i.e., ulcerative colitis and Crohn's disease) has been questionable. Omega-3 fat (fish oil) may delay a relapse in individuals with Crohn's disease, but otherwise appears to have no significant positive impact on inflammatory bowel disease.[34]

The following are general recommendations for feeding a healthy intestinal tract:

- Include yogurt with live bacteria, especially after taking antibiotics.
- Include fish (particularly fatty fish), especially if you have Crohn's disease.
- Include vegetables and fruits every day.

▨ CANCER RISK REDUCTION

The role of food in preventing as well as causing cancer is a hotly debated topic. Because most cancers take a long time to develop, studies to determine cause and effect are difficult and costly to conduct. Animal studies and laboratory experiments fuel many of the theories about the food and cancer relationship.

The relative amount of omega-3 to omega-6 fats in the diet has been implicated in the development of cancer. There is evidence from animal studies and population studies that fat may stimulate tumor development and growth. Higher intakes of omega-6 fats (from foods such as vegetables oils) increased breast tumors in animal studies.[35]

Table 7.7   Examples of Phytochemicals and Food Sources[36]

Phytochemicals	Food Sources
Anthocyanidins	Berries, such as blueberries, blackberries, raspberries, strawberries, and elderberries; red grapes; black-eyed peas; red cabbage; radishes; cherries; nuts, such as almonds, hazelnuts, pecans, and pistachios; cinnamon
Beta-cryptoxanthine	Citrus fruit, papayas, and pumpkin
Flavan-3-ols	Black tea; green tea; red wine; dark chocolate
Flavanones	Citrus fruit, such as lemons, limes, oranges, tangerines, and grapefruit
Flavones	Parsley
Flavonols	Arugula, kale, okra, onion, and peas
Isoflavones	Soy products, such as soy beans, edamame, soy burgers, miso, natto, soy cheese, soy milk, soy flour, tofu, soy nuts, tempeh, and soy yogurt
Lutein + zeaxanthin	Broccoli, carrots, green leafy vegetables, and pumpkin
Lycopene	Cooked tomatoes, pink grapefruit, and watermelon

Source: U.S. Department of Agriculture, Agricultural Research Service. Nutrient Data Laboratory Web site: http://www.ars.usda.gov/nutrientdata.

The Seven Countries Study and the Lyon Diet Heart Study both showed a low rate of cancer as well as heart disease in this population who consumed a "Mediterranean diet," that is a diet rich in fish and omega-3 fat (as opposed to omega-6 fat).[37]

Phytochemicals in foods may reduce the risk of cancer although the way(s) this occurs remains elusive. Theories include protecting DNA from damage and mutation, stimulating death of abnormal cells, and preventing the growth of new blood vessels, thus cutting off nutrients and oxygen from the cancerous lesion. All of these hypotheses have yet to be proven in studies of humans.

While specific and definitive dietary recommendations have varied with regard to cancer risk reduction, certain general recommendations can be made:

- Choose the fats in your diet wisely.
- Limit total and saturated fat intake.

- Include vegetables and fruits every day.
- Include fish (particularly fatty fish).
- Include nuts several times per week.
- Maintain a healthy weight.

▨ DIET AND LONGEVITY

Can the foods I eat add years to my life? There have been some studies that have explored this. Researchers in the EPIC (European Prospective Investigation into Cancer and Nutrition) study[38] recruited over 74,000 men and women in nine European countries who were healthy and at least 60 years old. The researchers rated their diets using a traditional Mediterranean diet as the standard. The Mediterranean diet is rich in produce, legumes, whole grains, and fish, with limited amounts of red meat and saturated fat. Those study participants with diets most closely resembling the Mediterranean diet had a significantly longer life expectancy.

Longevity may also be positively impacted by a low meat diet. A review of six studies suggested that a low meat or vegetarian eating style increased longevity, with a 3.6 year increase for individuals who had been vegetarians for 20 or more years.[39]

More controversial has been the use of calorie-restricted diets to increase life span. In numerous animal studies, limiting food intake has resulted in life spans greater than would be expected for the species studied. How these findings relate to humans remains to be determined. One experiment, the CALERIE Study,[40] looked at biological markers of aging in a small group of healthy adults whose calorie intake was restricted. In one group, calories were reduced by 25 percent from their baseline or normal requirements, while in a second group, calories were reduced by 12.5 percent and energy expenditure via exercise was increased by 12.5 percent. A third group received a very low calorie diet of less than 900 calories per day. The study lasted six months. Two markers of aging, fasting insulin level and body temperature, did decrease by the end of the study suggesting that calorie restriction, whether by food reduction or a combination of food reduction and increased physical activity, might increase longevity. However, larger and longer studies are needed before this conclusion can be drawn. In addition, one must consider the ramifications of restrictive eating in terms of meeting nutrient needs. The less we eat, the more critical are our food choices to ensure vitamins, minerals, appropriate fats, sufficient fiber, and the host of phytochemicals necessary to keep our bodies in top form.

PUTTING IT ALL TOGETHER

> Above all, try something
>
> –FDR

If asked to distill the dietary recommendations listed above into a simplified plan, it would appear to be simple and not terribly novel or exciting:

- Eat at least 4–5 servings of fruits and 4–5 servings of vegetables each day.
- Choose unrefined grains and grain products most of the time.
- Include fish, especially fatty fish, at least twice each week.
- Have 2–3 servings of low-fat or fat-free dairy products each day.
- Choose monounsaturated fat–rich foods, but go easy on portions.
- Include nuts and seeds each week, as condiments rather than snacks.
- Keep well hydrated, choosing water over other beverages.

As simple as these recommendations are, most adults in the United States fall far short of them. When we add in the "fine-tuning" for health and wellness concerns noted previously, the task becomes that much more challenging. Knowledge does not equal action, and it is action that is needed to live stronger and live longer.

So, make this journey at your own pace. To start, choose one small and easy-to-make change in your diet, and practice it. As this change becomes incorporated into your daily routine, add another new behavior or food choice. With time, patience, and perseverance, your good health and vigor will reflect your improved choices. And, if there are times when you are struggling, remember that this is a journey and we are all a work in progress.

8

Impact of Lifestyle on Health

ANNA C. FREITAG, M.D., F.A.C.P., F.A.C.E., F.A.C.D.S.

The greatest reward of being a physician is helping people overcome illness and disability, restoring them to good health, and saving and prolonging the quality of their lives. As an endocrinologist, I have the opportunity not only to treat diseases, but also to assist in their prevention.

Modern science has changed the way we think about the world, including aging. Overwhelming research now indicates that lifestyles influence our health and longevity far more than had been believed in the past. Medical advances and healthier lifestyles have made living past the age of 50 more rewarding. Extended longevity used to be the exclusive domain of science fiction; however, with the quantum leaps that have been made in medicine and science, we are, for the first time in history, seeing the possibility of controlling one's health and life span.

In order to plan for a longer and healthier life, I would like to introduce you to a new phrase that is becoming a symbol of modern preventive medicine: self-induced diseases. As we know, a healthy lifestyle reduces the risk of ill health, while careless living clearly leads to an array of symptoms that can develop into a disease, sometimes of a chronic nature.

To a large extent, our choices determine the quality of our health and longevity. For example, we know that cigarette smoking, substance abuse, exposure to sun, improper diet, obesity, and a sedentary lifestyle are factors that contribute to the development of diseases; yet, millions of people do choose to indulge in these activities regardless of the consequences.

Statistical evidence clearly shows that an unhealthy lifestyle is harmful to our health, so what are we waiting for? It is time for change!

A doctor's goal is to reduce self-induced diseases in the twenty-first century by medical resources as well as by informing patients about their bodies' functioning.

■ ■ ■

The *endocrine, immune, and nervous systems* are known as the three master controls of the body. If any one of these systems is not working well, modern medicine can trace the origin of a disease that, when diagnosed at an early stage, may be prevented and treated successfully.

As an endocrinologist, I see, on a daily basis, how the *endocrine system* profoundly impacts every organ in the body.

- Insulin produced by the pancreas controls sugar levels in the body. It can be secreted in excess, in genetically predisposed persons, in response to eating sugars and carbohydrates and thereby contribute to weight gain, a precursor mechanism involved in the development of type 2 diabetes.
- The thyroid hormone, produced by the thyroid gland, has receptors all over the body and controls metabolism.
- Cortisol made by the adrenal gland is necessary for all essential body functions, including anti-inflammation, and response to physical and emotional stress.
- The estrogen and progesterone hormones in women are made by the ovaries in response to the follicle-stimulating hormone and the lutenizing hormone released by the pituitary gland; analogously in men, testosterone is made by the testes.
- Lepin and adiponectin are made by adipose fat tissue to indicate satiety and inhibit appetite.
- Vasopressin, produced by the posterior pituitary gland, allows us to concentrate our urine.

Having a healthy endocrine system may prevent the onset of many medical conditions before they become disabling diseases. How well we care for our bodies, including what we eat, how well we sleep, monitor stress levels, and oxygenize the body, impacts our general health and longevity.

The second master control, the *immune system,* monitors our health. When an organ is under attack by viruses, bacteria, or fungi, the immune system finds the intruders, makes the antibodies against them, and destroys them. As we age, the immune system slows down and sometimes fails to block dangerous invader cells that permit genetic mutations, allowing cancer or infection to replicate in the body.

Cancer is a typical disease related to a deficiency of the immune system and therefore is much more prevalent in the elderly; however, it tends to grow slower in older persons as compared to younger adults, who more often will manifest the highly malignant and fast-growing cancers.

Pneumonia or a urinary tract infection, when left untreated, often leads to the death of the senior with a slowed immune system. The infections can easily lead to sepsis, affecting the body system. What can be done to boost the immune system?

- Proper nutrition is a priority for a healthy body.
- Trans fats, refined carbohydrates, and salt should be consumed in moderation.
- Eat an abundance of fresh fruits and vegetables.
- Include two 3–4 ounce portions of protein per day.
- Decrease stress.
- Oxygenate the body. Deeply inhale fresh air.
- Eliminate toxins, such as smoking, alcohol, and environmental poisons.

The *nervous system* is the third master control of the body. Nerve conduction velocity is an important factor that measures a person's capacity to respond to stimuli. This tends to slow down with aging mainly because the brain dendrites conducting impulses to cells in the body are hardening.

The brain is the number one ''use-it-or-lose-it'' organ. You need to exercise your brain with the same vigor as your muscles, thereby creating new brain connections that improve nerve conduction velocity and memory. To exercise your nervous system and keep it healthy, I recommend any of the following activities:

- learn new skills,
- read,
- engage in mental activity and stimulation (play games, do crossword puzzles, and so forth),

- exercise (oxygenate the brain),
- eat a proper diet, including supplements of omega-3 fatty acids (at least 1,000 mg per day),
- minimize stress and maximize positive thinking,
- socialize; isolation leads to mental deterioration.

As a rule, what is good for your heart is good for your brain and vice versa. Positive thinking influences your cells and will reinforce your health.

Your eyes are an integral part of your nervous system. I recommend annual ophthalmologic exams for anyone suffering from diabetes, hypertension, or cardiovascular disease as these conditions sometimes present themselves in the eyes, can gradually damage the tiny blood vessels of the eyes and retina, and can accelerate the formation of cataracts.

■ ■ ■

In addition to the three master controls of the body, there are very important parts of the body's structure that are dependent on our well-being.

Muscle mass tends to reduce with age, even for the most avid athlete. This gradual decline actually starts in the late 20s or early 30s. Most people lose only about 1 percent of their muscle mass per year—women more than men. The less active you are, the faster your muscle will atrophy. So, use it or lose it! Lifting weights can increase muscle mass even in persons more than 80–90 years old. (I suggest consulting a personal trainer to minimize risk of injury if embarking on any new exercise regimen.)

Bones become brittle with age, more so for women than men because of postmenopausal estrogen losses as well as hormones, which play a critical role in sustaining strong bodies. However, a lack of vitamin D in the American diet and avoidance of sunlight can create low bone density in both sexes. Low bone density can be reversed at any age by

- adding more calcium-rich food to your diet: dairy products, vegetables, and fruits;
- avoiding smoking, drinking carbonated beverages, as well as excessive alcohol, all of which are clearly associated with bone loss;
- doing weight-bearing exercise, which has been shown to reverse bone loss and also helps to maintain bone mass; and

- moderate exposure to the sun, which can replenish vitamin D. Or, one can choose to take a vitamin D supplement of at least 400 I.U. (international units) per day (which also proves to boost the immune system and support healthy blood vessels).

Arthritis is a typical example of a wear-and-tear condition, which occurs in more than 100 forms. It is caused by the deterioration of cartilage between bone and joints. While medication reduces arthritic pain, the condition itself can be minimized with a proper diet, weight control, and regular exercise.

I recommend low-impact exercise in lieu of high-impact activities, such as walking instead of jogging, lifting lighter weights with increased repetitions, and lifting heavier weights more slowly. The goal is to develop the muscles above and below the joint, thereby relieving pressure on the joint.

We often hear that we need to accept and love our bodies. I do believe that we should love our essence, but not necessarily our bad habits and addictions, which can ruin our health, undermine longevity, and deprive us of independence in our senior years. I am referring to the causes of self-induced diseases.

Diabetes is a textbook example of a self-induced disease that is rampant today in adults, adolescents, and even children. It is caused by the high fat and sodium diet found in fast foods, trans-fatty acids (abundant in processed "junk" food), and inactivity. There is a clear and direct correlation between obesity and diabetes. Excessive eating habits are a way of "medicating" oneself for unresolved psychological problems. Self-indulgence is more important to people than self-preservation.

The incidence of type 2 diabetes tends to coincide with slower metabolic rates and decreasing mobility; therefore, it is more frequent in seniors who move less with increasing age. Fortunately, diabetics have many choices in managing the disease, and potential diabetics now have a multitude of options for weight loss and prevention.

- Regardless of age, exercise or changes in diet have helped many to change their lifestyles and control food consumption rather than be controlled by it.
- Bolstering the endocrine system is essential for increased health. Consumption of healthier foods, such as fruits, vegetables, and grains, produces visible results. A serving size of meat or fish should be no larger than the palm of your hand.

- Avoid sweetened beverages such as soda, excessive consumption of juice, caffeinated drinks, and alcohol, including wine and beer.
- Keep physically active. Exercise or walk on a regular basis. Start slowly and build up to 30 minutes of aerobic exercise daily. If you prefer, you can take at least 5,000 steps per day, as measured by a pedometer.
- Lift weights: Start with ½-lb weights, gradually increasing the amount of weight as strength increases. Strengthening the upper body tends to improve posture, which, in turn, increases metabolism and burns more calories (even at rest).
- Impact sports, such as basketball, should be played against people of your own age and fitness group. It is recommended that you obtain cardiovascular clearance from your physician before embarking on any new exercise regime.

Controlling diabetes, hypertension, and hypercholesterolemia can greatly minimize much of their associated pathology, such as micro- and macrovascular flow to the brain, eyes, kidneys, nervous system, extremities, and gastrointestinal tract.

Addiction to prescription drugs is of no small importance. Thousands of books have been written about addiction to drugs and its consequences. Billions have been spent to eradicate addiction to illegal drugs. A war was declared on substance abuse by former U.S. Secretary of Health, Education, and Welfare Joseph A. Califano Jr., who continues to fight against this social problem of major proportions. The recent deaths of many prominent personalities in sports, the arts, and corporate life highlight the extent of this serious problem. American model Anna Nicole Smith and popular actor Heath Ledger both died at a young age following drug overdose. Dependency on prescription drugs is also known as "performance dependency." When people cannot achieve their expected goals as set by ambition, they often turn to drugs to bolster energy levels, thereby creating a health hazard. Overdosing on legal or illegal drugs is a frequent occurrence.

While medication may temporarily help performance levels, continued use for this purpose is detrimental to health. The recent deaths of Anna Nicole Smith and her son illustrate the danger of prescription drugs if they are not coordinated among varied physicians and the body is exposed to conflicting chemical reactions.

As the patient, you are responsible for informing your physicians about any medication you are using, including vitamins, herbs, or other supplements. Providing a written list of all current medications and their doses is the best way to inform your doctors as well as pharmacist in order to avoid drug interaction. For example, some medications cannot be taken with milk, while others do not mix with other foods.

If you take a prescribed performance-enhancing medication, you should make sure to get plenty of rest and oxygenize your body by practicing yoga, meditation, or any other form of relaxation techniques.

If your stress is relationship related, you should consult a professional to help reduce or eliminate the triggers that cause stress.

Cigarette smoking is also a major health hazard and a contributor to lung cancer. Still, millions of individuals, addicted to nicotine, are unwilling to give up this destructive habit, which can lead to many self-induced diseases and death. Nicotine addicts ''medicate'' themselves by smoking in order to avoid dealing with underlying problems, thus perpetuating dependence on cigarettes.

New efficient drugs and programs are providing various means for the cessation of smoking, such as Zyban and Commit Lozenges, and most hospitals now provide group smoking cessation classes. Dependency on nicotine should be coordinated with psychological counseling, so that regression to smoking is permanently blocked.

Coronary disease is the number one killer in the United States. Stroke and heart disease are oftentimes called the ''executive diseases'' because they affect, to a large extent, individuals that have high-powered, stressful positions in corporate life.

The successful executive may find it difficult to change his or her lifestyle due to the high-level of competition that accompanies such success. However, in spite of the fact that stress is a trademark of corporate life, it is possible to reduce the likelihood of sudden casualties. Here are my recommendations for preventing potential coronary disease:

- You are what you eat, and you can imagine your food as if it floats around in your bloodstream. I recommend that you eat more vegetables, fruit, and fiber and drink lots of water. Eating fibrous foods and drinking water will help to flush out your kidneys and gastrointestinal tract of impurities. Some branded diets that I recommend include The South Beach Diet and the DASH (Dietary Approaches to Stop Hypertension) Diet.
- Perform a cardiovascular exercise of approximately 30 minutes a day in order to work your heart. Consider consulting a personal trainer.

- Take one coated baby aspirin (81 mg) per day for persons at risk, if there are no contraindications in doing so.
- Practice yoga for relaxation: 30–60 minutes. Most heart attacks and strokes occur between the hours of 6:00 A.M. and 9:00 A.M. because of the increased pulse and blood pressure at this time of day, which correlates with surges in serum cortisol and catecholamines (adrenaline).
- Meditation has a calming effect, slows down your heart rate, and lowers your blood pressure. There is evidence that this behavior change can make a huge difference in overall cardiovascular health and ultimate longevity.
- Body massage is also a great stress reducer.

Clearly cardiovascular problems increase with age, most especially in the sedentary adult. This is mainly due to hypertension, atherosclerosis, and hyperlipidemia, which need to be tightly controlled to minimize their devastating complications to the heart, brain, kidneys, and other organs.

With today's noninvasive technology such as the ultrafast CT (computed tomography) angiograms of the coronary arteries, we can look at all of our coronary blood vessels. This technology did not exist a decade ago. Also available are medications that stop and can even reverse the production of atherosclerotic plaque. I agree with leaders in the field of cardiology who believe that a heart attack can be prevented.

The *environmental impact* on health is much more prevalent and serious than is generally believed.

Millions of people are ''roasting'' in the hot sun on beaches, ignoring the danger of skin cancer, degeneration of the macula, and opacification of the lens in the eyes, increase in glaucoma, suppression of the immune system, and other conditions. Skin cancer can lead to melanoma that can cause death if not diagnosed early.

The leading cause of cataracts is long-term sun exposure. Minimizing sun exposure and wearing sunglasses that block out 400 UVB (ultraviolet light B) are highly advisable. Fortunately, today, doctors can easily manage and fix cataracts, glaucoma, and even problems with focus, and new treatments are emerging for macular degeneration.

While excessive exposure to the sun is detrimental, some exposure to the sun during the winter months is helpful in the prevention and treatment of seasonal affective disorder, or SAD, which is a result of insufficient exposure to light. SAD is experienced as a depressive state, and a decrease in symptoms usually coincides with increased intensity of light in the spring.

Also, vitamin D deficiency can be prevented with only 10–15 minutes of sun exposure per day. Not only is vitamin D essential for healthy bones, but it is now considered important for cardiovascular health and the immune system.

Radon is a hazardous environmental gas that can cause various types of cancer in an otherwise healthy person. This odorless, radioactive gas, produced by decay of radium in rocks and soil, penetrates into houses that are built in rocky areas and causes gradual but fatal damage to an organism. Everybody should have their dwellings tested for the presence of this gas.

▪ ▪ ▪

One of the most frequently asked questions is, "What determines life span?" Scientists have been attempting to answer this complex question for decades. If we knew what precipitates aging, we could prevent the latent changes within the body that lead to its ultimate decline. Thus far, the best explanation is provided by the concept known as the "Hayflick limit."

In 1986, Dr. Leonard Hayflick and Dr. Paul Morehead demonstrated that cells do have a limited capacity for renewal. They can repair themselves when they are worn or damaged, but cannot regenerate more than 52 times. Dr. Hayflick and Dr. Morehead's findings raise a fundamental question: If cells renew themselves on the average only 52 times, why do people who were born during the same year die at different times?

Let me answer this intriguing question: Inside every human cell are telomeres, segments of DNA that are located on the end of chromosomes. A telomere is an important biomarker that automatically shortens its tail as we age. We could theoretically stop the aging process if we could prolong the telomere's end. On the end of the telomere there is an enzyme called telomerase that lengthens the telomere's tail and regenerates it, but gradually becomes inactive. The issue is how to increase the activity of telomerase and, thus, how to extend the telomere's tail. The increase in the telomerase activity is related to the mitochondrion that has its own DNA, inherited solely from the mother. The mitochondrion provides enzymes with the essential energy to generate the nucleotide ATP (adenosine triphosphate), which influence the extension of the telomerase.

However, we are not passive participants in the biological determinism. A healthy lifestyle may influence how quickly the 52 cellular cycles renew. Bodies with high wear and tear, suppressed immune systems, or clogged metabolic channels, among other conditions, clearly call for faster cellular renewal than organisms whose cells have lesser demand for repair. The time span between the deaths of twins, born at the same time and from the same stock genetically, demonstrates that the Hayflick limit can be slowed down by our individual input—making our health a priority.

Recent research at Harvard Medical School, by Dr. David Sinclair and Dr. Christoph Westphal, has shown that sirtuins, a newly discovered class of enzymes that control aging in rodents, mimic the beneficial effects of longevity of calorie restriction and exercise and influence eating habits. Activating these enzymes seems to dramatically increase the life span of the rodents. This and many other experiments, which aim at improving health and extending longevity, are paving the way for a future when aging will be a pleasure.

You may be wondering why I am elaborating on these details that do not appear to be relevant to your daily routine. The reason is that to a large extent, only you determine how these 75 trillion cells in your body will function. You can control what you eat, how you oxygenize your body, monitor the level of stress, and protect yourself from pollutants. You have the power to greatly influence the quality of health and well-being in your senior years.

I have tried to stress that we can either prevent or self-induce diseases. Understanding the extraordinary complexity of the human body will increase your awareness that you are not the helpless victim of what "your genetics do to you," but rather that your thoughts and your mind are powerful allies that can determine the quality of your health.

We now consider the span of middle age to be approximately from 40 to 65 years of age. The great news is that most people between 50 and 75 years of age are much healthier than were people of the same age group 30 years ago.

The onset of diseases can be prevented with effort, determination, a healthy diet, regular exercise, and the elimination of vices, such as smoking and excessive alcohol consumption. If people invest time and energy into healthy living, I strongly believe they will be rewarded by a quality of life that will be worth the investment.

Today's preoccupation with staying young stems from the necessity to stay independent longer. However, the question is not only how do we live longer, but also how do we make our longer lives healthier. Recent studies indicate that genetic factors determine only about 35 percent of one's ultimate mortality. Most of one's destiny is under one's own control. If seniors are given "instructions" on how to keep themselves healthier longer and they follow the guidelines so that their organs regenerate, they can reverse the aging process. I do believe that in our lifetime, we will see the promise of stem cells and genetic engineering's ability to tailor-make individualized medicine, which will add quality years to our lives.

My intent in writing this chapter is to empower seniors through information to make more positive decisions to prevent self-induced diseases and enjoy longer and better lives.

9

Modern Medicine and Rejuvenation

JOEL B. SINGER, M.D., F.A.C.S.

We have all done it—stood in front of the mirror examining every perceived "fault" on our faces and bodies.

Our appearances can have immense influence in how we treat ourselves and how we are treated by others. If we are unhappy with some of our features, our self-perception can adversely affect us. It has been demonstrated that the physical changes produced by cosmetic surgery have positive psychological effects. People who have undergone cosmetic surgery often display renewed energy, an increase in self-confidence, and become more outgoing socially. These positive changes hold true regardless of age, race, or gender. We all want to feel good about ourselves and be accepted by others. This is particularly true when our bodies are aging and we still need to be professionally competitive or socially desirable.

When cosmetic products are no longer sufficient to cover the aging epidermis or sagging muscles, it is time to consider medical evaluation and procedures. Corrective surgeries of all kinds continue to be developed rapidly because of ongoing improvements in technology as well as innovative techniques and procedures. In the past, beautification was the domain of women, but, with increasing longevity and the need to extend professional activities far beyond the age of 65, men are frequently seeking the expertise of plastic surgeons to keep a competitive appearance with younger men.

If you consider a consultation with a plastic surgeon, the first step is to make sure that he or she has the proper credentials:

- First, inquire whether the doctor has certification in plastic surgery and not some other medical specialty. If in doubt, contact the American Board of Medical Specialties.
- Find out whether the doctor has proper training in the areas that you are considering. How many procedures has he or she performed before you?
- Does the doctor have photos of before and after results from previous procedures, so that you can judge the results of his or her expertise?
- If the procedure is performed in the doctor's office, make sure there is a proper operating room suite, licensed by the state, with a staff able to assist during the operation and appropriately certified anesthesia providers.
- Get a written statement about the cost of the procedure, including payment options.
- How long will the surgery take?
- Postoperative conditions vary. Find out how long you will be unable to go to work or be limited in activities.

There is an array of procedures ranging from surgical to nonsurgical interventions. I will review them and comment on their specific features so that you may decide which of them would be appropriate for you. For some, correcting the contours of the body is essential to enhance a youthful appearance; for others, even a minor change on the face may produce a positive outcome. Beyond the frequently used procedures for beautification, there are also many reconstructive surgeries that I will not mention, such as enhancement of an undeveloped chin or flat cheeks, that are custom-made on demand by specialized reconstructive surgeons.

As seniors are reaching a more advanced age than ever before, they not only want to live longer, but also healthier and younger. Cosmetic surgery is giving many of them the chance to rejuvenate: Roughly 7.5 million Americans improve their appearances each year with some form of plastic surgery.

While considering cosmetic surgery, a person should be clear about the motivations for the improvement. For some, improvement in appearance is a needed trigger to begin a different lifestyle; for others, such as actors or other performers, it is a professional necessity. Seniors who are intellectually younger than their chronological ages need to balance their inner youth with their improved appearances. Whatever the reason for plastic surgery intervention, the procedure will not change who you are internally.

▥ SURGICAL PROCEDURES

The plastic surgeries for improvement of face and body include the following specialties:

Breast lifts (mastopexy) do not enlarge the breasts; the procedure lifts only the upper part of the breasts. Following the surgery, the vast majority of women retain their enhanced, more youthful-looking breasts for years without any further surgical intervention.

Breast augmentation (augmentation mammoplasty) modifies the size and the shape of the breasts. The procedure can be performed in two to three hours and on an outpatient basis. The benefits of breast augmentation include uniformly sized breasts, enlarged breasts by one or two sizes, or reconstruction of breasts altered by prior surgery. Visible scarring varies from patient to patient, but the skin tone around the incision eventually returns to normal, and scarring becomes minimal. Most people are able to resume normal activities within a few days after the surgery.

Breast reduction (reduction mammoplasty) is usually done when the size of the breasts causes discomfort, skin irritation, or difficulty to find clothing that properly fits the individual. Most women reported that the results from the breast reduction are so favorable that the concern about scarring is minimal. The surgery takes about two hours.

Eyelift surgery (blepharoplasty) removes excess fat, skin, and muscle along the upper or lower eyelids, resulting in a younger appearance. The eyelid surgery corrects drooping of the upper eyelids, puffy bags below the eyes, or corrects vision problems caused by drooping eyelids over the eye. It also erases crow's feet. The surgery is usually performed on an outpatient basis.

Face-lift surgery (rhytidectomy) is designed to remove the visible signs of aging, such as excess fat from the face and neck and drapes in the facial skin, and tighten sagging facial muscles. The surgery will not make you look like someone else or stop the aging process, but it will make you look younger.

Liposuction is performed when the goal is to remove unwanted fat from the abdomen, thighs, upper arms, chin, cheeks, or other fat tissues. The surgeon injects fluid into the fat tissue and suctions out the fat along with the fluid. Liposuction is recommended when dieting and exercise do not produce the desired results.

Surgical hair enhancement or **hair transplants** involve the removal of tiny hair follicles from hairy parts of the body or scalp and then implanting them into the balding area.

A **"weekend lift"** is a popular facial procedure involving minimal incisions, facial muscle tightening, and neck suspension with a special suture.

■ NONSURGICAL PROCEDURES

There are many products that can be injected to reduce the appearance of wrinkles and increase the youthful look:

Botox is a popular treatment known under the name of botulinum toxin, which is FDA (U.S. Food and Drug Administration) approved for cosmetic use. This product temporarily blocks nerve impulses to the muscle and prevents them from contracting, thus preventing creasing. Treatment is recommended for healthy men and women who need to eliminate outward symptoms of aging, including crow's feet, frown lines, forehead creases, or thick bands on the front of the neck. Botox reduces lines, but the results depend on skin elasticity, muscle responsiveness, and general health.

Restylane and **Juraderm** injections are now more popular than collagen because they last longer and do not require pretreatment skin tests. When injected, they produce results similar to botox treatment.

Fat injections are frequently used in patients who are concerned that they might develop an allergic reaction to a foreign substance (i.e., botox or restylane). First, liposuction is performed on a part of the body where there is residue of unwanted fat. The same fat is then promptly injected into an area where it eliminates wrinkles or enhances lips.

Chemical peels have been performed for several decades. This method improves skin on the face, neck, or chest. A chemical solution is applied to the skin, causing regeneration of the skin. Peels frequently reduce or eliminate fine lines around the eyes; however, deeper wrinkles do not respond to this type of treatment. After the peel, the new skin is more sensitive to the environmental impact and may develop swelling, blisters, or crusting that lasts up to two to three weeks after the procedure.

Photofacials are another high-tech intervention: The IPL, or intense pulsed light therapy, is FDA approved and requires about six sessions to achieve desired results. The benefits include elimination of dark aging spots, superficial capillaries, and diminishment of wrinkles. This method is also used for dermatologic conditions, such as rosacea or some types of dermatitis.

Laser resurfacing is a method used to resurface the outer layers of skin. High intensity laser light removes the superficial layer of skin, thus reducing wrinkles. New lasers using fractionated beams can achieve great results without a prolonged recovery. The achieved improvement lasts for years.

Microdermabrasion is a popular procedure that repairs facial skin by sandblasting it with tiny crystals and vacuuming the debris. It is a painless procedure that does not require recovery time; however, the benefits last only a few months.

▪ MEDICATED CREAMS

While the FDA regulates the safety of skin-care products, it is not responsible for their effectiveness. A variety of reactions exists in response to cosmetic products, depending on many factors, such as age, flexibility of skin, environmental damage, individual allergies, and general health.

The principal goal of a product is to activate the production of collagen that, with aging, is reduced and removes the outer layers of dead skin to accelerate new layers of epidermis to appear. Chemicals or vitamin C in a concentrated form achieves the abrasion of the skin. Hydrating creams are needed to provide missing moisture to the skin that was depleted by abrasion.

While staying young is the goal of increasing numbers of men and women, cosmetic surgery is not the only way to achieve it. Seniors need to become informed customers on the market of rejuvenation approaches in order to decide what the best choice is for them in hopes of living a quality life.

My recommendations for the extension of a quality life would include the following "musts":

- Develop a pattern of sleep that regenerates your energy.
- Keep physically and mentally active.
- Choose your diet carefully because it determines your appearance to a large extent.
- Oxygenize your body by exercise or walking every day, health permitting.
- Avoid smoking, the use of excessive amounts of drugs, and exposure to the sun.

- Keep a positive view of your past, present, and future. A glass is always half full or half empty; choose to see it half full on the way to fulfillment.
- Avoid stressful events and relationships if you can. There are many strategies to do that and qualified professionals can help you to organize your life and declutter it from unwanted weight.
- Have a purpose in life, no matter how small. Individuals with a purpose live longer, happier lives. Nothing boosts a better appearance and better health than happiness and contentment from doing something good for others.

Youthful appearance is not only a matter of rejuvenating intervention—it is also a matter of lifestyle. Develop in your mind a picture of the self, how you would like to look and live as if you have already reached your desired goal. We know that our thoughts have a much greater impact on our actions and behavior than we realize. Thus, seeing yourself as progressing toward the ideal self will help you to achieve your goal faster.

I have practiced plastic surgery for over 30 years and know that even a small improvement can have a great impact on a person's self-image. When I meet with a new patient, I do not see a single part of the body that needs to be corrected. I see the whole person and cooperate with the new candidate on the selection of the best possible and most affordable method to achieve the maximum possible effects.

Remember that you are the one who has a "dream." With their expertise, doctors are here to assist you in order to help you move closer to your goals.

10 ▪ ▪ ▪

Fitness at 50 and Beyond

It is a paradox that after being physically active all our lives we have
to exercise to stay physically fit.

Tom Collingwood, Ph.D.
Robert Carkuff, Ph.D.

The importance of physical fitness will take on a new significance in the
twenty-first century. In the 1980s, public awareness of the beneficial
impact of exercise on health and longevity started a boom that has
grown during the past 25 years into a culture of awareness among
health-conscious individuals. What was initially a recreational activity
and fun is now becoming a solution to health problems on a national
level. It is timely to highlight this new phenomenon and its importance
for seniors.

The graying of America, or the demographic of aging, is a continuous
process that impacts the national economy and public health in a much
greater way than we realize.[1] In order to secure for us and our children a
life in a healthy and economically stable society, our government must
regulate demographic changes to prevent the excess of ill, aging people
whose medical and retirement needs could imbalance the ratio between
the working and the dependent segment of the society. As an increasing
number of baby boomers are beginning to retire, the need to keep
the population young, fit, and working longer is becoming of major
importance.[2] It is vital to realize that the elderly will increase in most
countries during the next 50 years, and we need to be prepared for the

consequences of such growth that will have an impact on health policy as well as on the social and the economic reality of people in the United States.[3]

In order to maintain the health of an aging population at the best possible level, we need to address the national increase in obesity, not only among the elderly, but also in younger people. Obesity is recognized as a national health problem of major proportions that can cause many disabling diseases such as diabetes, heart disease, damage to internal organs, and also may lead to gradual helplessness and loss of productivity.

One of the major reasons for the increase of obesity, besides food, is a sedentary lifestyle exacerbated by technology that reduces physical activities to a minimum. Where our ancestors walked, we drive a car; where they climbed the stairs, we use the elevators; machines do the work for us, and our interests in sports gravitate from practicing them to watching athletes on the television.[4] The human body is missing the activity for which it was built. This fact alone highlights the importance of physical activity as an obesity fighter.

Dr. Roy J. Shephard states in his book *Aging, Physical Activity, and Health* that 57 percent of elderly men and 63 percent of women who applied for life insurance had a body mass 10 percent or more above the actuarial limits.[5] The U.S. population between the ages of 24 and 74 was reported overweight. African American women had 48.7 percent higher prevalence of obesity than Caucasian women who reached 34.0 percent.[6] Paradoxically, the prevalence of overweight individuals was higher among those living below the poverty level.

As already mentioned in previous chapters, genes influence only about 25 to 30 percent of our development, while the major impact on health depends on our lifestyles. Since obesity is a self-induced condition, we may reduce or eliminate it by controlling our diets and activities. Numerous studies confirm that physical exercise can counterbalance the detrimental effect of a sedentary life on health. If we do not make 5,000 steps per day, our health may suffer. Anyone who by choice or professional necessity is bound to a sedentary existence should wear a pedometer and check the number of steps at the end of each day. If the minimum is not attained, walking on a treadmill or outdoors may be considered.[7] Achieving 10,000 steps per day results almost immediately in a better sleep pattern, increased energy, vigor, improvement in digestive irregularities, and elimination of varied pains.

If the body is left to its own development, it annually diminishes by about 1 percent. By age 60, people have lost on the average about 10 to 20 percent of their maximum strength. However, this physiological finding is not reflected by the population at large. Some seniors are strong, energetic, and flexible, while others of the same age are weaker, less vigorous, and rigid.[8] It is in our own interests to be informed about the causes of such differences.

Physical decline that usually accompanies aging does not have to happen to us. We have the means to prevent it to a very large extent if we have the will. Exercise is one of the magical "pills" for sustaining not only our youth and vigor, but also our health. Physicians often recognize the value of exercise and recommend walking or other sports to prevent cardiovascular risk, to increase pulmonary performance, to reduce weight and hypertension, and to alleviate other conditions. We should be aware that physical activities are only an adjunct to medical treatment and never the sole remedy.

We also have to realize that occasional exercise will not accomplish much for our health, even though it is better than nothing. The key is to exercise daily and to select the type of activity that is appropriate for the goals we want to achieve.

▪ ▪ ▪

The surge of fitness centers during the past 20 years reflects the desire of the general public to fight signs of decline and aging by staying vigorous and healthy. The National Health Interview Survey estimates that enhancement of physical and mental activities will play a major role in sustaining an aging population to be independent, healthy, and able to contribute to society.[9] Dr. Herbert A. deVries, gerontologist from the University of Southern California, states that Americans in their 50s, 60s, 70s, 80s, and 90s will have more influence than any of their earlier contemporaries for setting the cultural, political, and economic tones of society.[10]

Are seniors ready for such a challenge? Extended longevity is not only an opportunity for longer and healthier lives, but also for the development of a purpose and new meaningful roles for seniors in shaping a new social order where they will not be dead wood, but rather participants in the revitalization of an evolving demography. Changes do not occur fast, but represent a process where new possibilities are considered and gradually practiced until they are integrated as an accepted way of life. The role of physical exercise in the lives of this generation is a change in process.

The University of California, known for its research in the field of gerontology, developed a program intended to test the effects of physical fitness on seniors. Two hundred men and women, aged 50 to 87 years, participated in varied physical activities ranging from walking, jogging, calisthenics, to static stretching and more. Volunteers were examined by a physician before the program started, and they also were tested during and after the exercises: Six weeks later, improvement had been reported in all of them. Their body fat decreased, oxygen capacity and strength increased, and symptoms of nervous tension, headaches, chronic back pain, constipation, and insomnia diminished or disappeared. Several participants reported increases in sexual activity. Moreover, mortality dropped among seniors who exercised and developed healthy lifestyles.[11]

It is rather surprising that in spite of repeated studies demonstrating the benefits of fitness programs for health, 49 million people in the United States are sedentary. The resistance to work for health was evident in a survey of 121 seniors in Connecticut: 86 percent reported that they are fit to walk to the shopping center, but almost 50 percent of the same individuals described themselves as "disabled" when asked whether they can walk for pleasure.[12]

Resistance to physical activities represents the atavistic conflict between the biological tendency and the higher awareness of self. Entropy pulls us down to stagnation and physiologic decline, while the spiritual self inspires us to overcome entropy by working toward health and fulfillment of our physical potentials. Exercise does not only reduce varied unwanted symptoms, but it can also increase self-esteem and joy when a desired goal is reached. Dr. Gary Small reports that working out may culminate in a sense of euphoria, referred to as the runner's high, which results from the stimulation of endorphins.[13]

Most people do not protect their bodies enough and tend to use and abuse them for external goals until they reach their breaking points. Sufficient mobility and oxygenation of an organism is one of the means to convey to our cells that we care. If we do not give the body what it deserves, it will give to us what we deserve: headaches and diseases.

Many seniors resist exercising because they erroneously believe that it will deprive them of energy. The opposite is true. A sedentary life and inactivity consume more energy than we realize.

■ ■ ■

When we start something new we want to succeed. When we plan a fitness program, we want to get back what we invested, or more.

The prerequisite for a successful fitness experience is to know what you want to accomplish. If you are not sure, look at yourself in the mirror, observe your posture and gait, and the movement of and balance of your body in motion. Check your sitting flexibility. Do you have difficulty getting out of a chair? Do you shuffle when you walk? Is your posture bent? Are your movements coordinated? The same scrutiny can be applied to enhancing your awareness of the internal state of the body.

Once you know what you want to improve, you either consult a trainer or decide yourself what kind of exercise will make a meaningful difference.

From the multitude of physical fitness models and techniques intended for people of all ages, we selected those that are most helpful for seniors. They are summarized in the following broad categories:

- exercising for weight loss;
- exercising to stay fit;
- exercising to stay young.

The above objectives can be reached by one or a mixture of techniques that are known in the fitness world as the three pillars of exercises:

- cardiovascular conditioning;
- strength and power training;
- flexibility and balance training.

Exercise for weight loss consists of a wide range of dynamic activities that are stimulating the metabolic rate and burning calories.

Cardiovascular and pulmonary conditioning boosts cardiovascular fitness as more oxygen enters the blood and improves the efficiency of the heart and the lungs. There are several popular exercises in this category:

- Aerobics are the favorite exercise of seniors who have medical clearance for vigorous activities. Aerobic means "not out of breath," which is a reminder that the heart rate should never exceed 65–75 beats at maximum.
- Walking is a superior way to lose weight. You may start with as little as five minutes daily, no excuses, and increase it gradually to one hour. Unfortunately, inclement weather may be a reason for not walking. We recommend installation of a treadmill in your home or office. Anytime you have a few minutes, you can walk. It is the frequency of practice that produces results.
- Swimming can be practiced indoors or outdoors. Besides having a beneficial effect on the heart, it stimulates the muscles and joints. An additional benefit is pool walking that can be practiced for about 15 minutes as a warm-up before swimming. This strengthens calfs, thighs, and also the torso.
- Cycling, practiced at home or outdoors, has a dual effect: It increases the cardiovascular system and strengthens the leg muscles. It is not recommended for those with pelvis or joint problems in the knees, dizzy spells, or unstable balance.
- Tennis and racquetball are competitive sports that are superior glycogen consumers. For a vigorous practice, a medical clearance is a must.
- Dancing is a great activity for a cardiovascular workout, as well as for balance and flexibility. For those who dance with joy and vigor, the performance can lead to a euphoric feeling that is similar to a runner's high.
- Nontraditional "sports": anyone who is involved in gardening or housework knows that these activities are proven fat burners. Raking or vacuuming, if done rhythmically, is an acceptable substitute for cardiovascular exercise.

An awareness of the metabolic changes that take place while we are exercising is crucial for increasing our conscious participation in the weight loss process. The key factor here is glycogen. This powerful polysaccharide is stored in the muscles, ready to empower the body with extra energy when it is in danger. It is used during exercising to booster the muscles and the heart. When the reserves are used, the body is replacing them. Our fatty molecules take action and replenish glycogen by absorbing glucose and proteins. If we lose 50 percent of glycogen, it will take 1 hour to rebuild 5 percent of the loss, or 10 hours to replenish it all.

The more often we exercise, the greater is the loss of glycogen and the more regular and intensive is the body's need to use available fatty cells and glucose. It explains why a person who is constantly on the go is slim, while the weight of a "couch potato" who has low mobility increases even with a reduced amount of food.

Calories are burned through invigorating the digestive system to constantly use fatty deposits that are clogging the cells. It is obvious that activities such as aerobics, brisk walking, jogging, bicycling, hiking, swimming, dancing, and similar motions are instrumental in reducing fats in the body. Women should give serious thought to reducing an excess of weight as more women than men die each year from heart disease; diabetic women have six times the risk of heart disease than nondiabetic women.

■ ■ ■

Exercise to stay fit: What does it mean to be fit? In general, it is the capacity for independent functioning in social, personal, and professional roles; physiologically, it is the amount of oxygen that the body receives and can use. The more oxygen the body uses, the more active it can be. Since the amount of oxygen that is carried around the blood stream depends on the functioning of the heart, unobstructed arteries and lung capacity need to interact flawlessly. Besides the exciting array of possibilities for cardiovascular conditioning already mentioned, we need to explore the practice of *strength and power training.*

Weight lifting, also known as pumping iron, or resistance training, strengthens muscles and increases their size and power. This exercise builds the body, protects joints, and decreases the pain of osteoarthritis.[14] For a home exercise, you will need a pair of dumbbells of three to five pounds each and an illustrated manual to follow the routine, or you may enroll in a fitness center and work with a trainer who will introduce you to a variety of equipment that will be suitable for your goals. Your age and strength are not factors in succeeding. Even seniors in their 90s benefit from weight lifting.

Dr. John W. Rowe and Dr. Robert L. Kahn refer to studies involving frail older people up to 98 years of age living in a long-term facility who were involved in a resistance training three times a week. On traditional equipment they exercised a routine that we print in its entity to demonstrate that seniors in their 10th decade not only completed the program, they enjoyed it, too:[15]

- bicep machine to strengthen upper arm muscles,
- shoulder exercise to strengthen upper arms and shoulders,

- knee extension to work quadriceps and thighs,
- triceps machine to strengthen muscles at the back,
- triceps machine II to strengthen upper arms,
- plantar flexors to strengthen the calfs,
- hip flexors to bring the knees toward the chest,
- hip abductors to strengthen muscles at the side of the hips, and
- hip extensors to strengthen the buttocks and lower back muscles.

The results were astounding. Those seniors who could not walk without assistance started to walk without canes. The results set in quickly, and the participants were able to retain their newfound functions with just one follow-up session per week. It is a myth that one cannot improve functioning because of old age. The MacArthur studies show that very old people who never have exercised are capable of becoming more physically fit.[16]

Flexibility of joints and balance training is intended to improve balance, increase the coordination of limbs, the flexibility of muscles, and provide oxygen to the blood and joints, allowing easier movement. As inactivity restricts the range of motion of joints, ligaments lose their flexibility. There are several choices in flexibility training:

- Pilates is an exercise concentrating on the strengthening of muscles of the stomach, buttocks, the lower back, and inner thighs. Some figures can be done on a mat; others require the assistance of an instructor and are done on special Pilate equipment. The benefit of the exercise is increased muscle strength and flexibility, better coordination, and improved balance.
- Yoga is a favored exercise consisting of poses and breathing exercises. It oxygenizes the body and increases blood flow to joints and muscles. It is essentially a relaxing exercise, reducing stiffness and stress.
- Tai chi consists of a series of slow movements that stretch and lengthen muscles and ligaments, increases breathing capacity, and improves balance. It is a favorable exercise of seniors because of its slow motion.

For a home exercise, it is helpful to have a trainer to help start the routine.

While selecting the best possible method or techniques for your rehabilitation or makeover objectives, we recommend three steps before you make a commitment.

- Whatever method or technique you select, it should be easy, fun, and nondisruptive to other daily activities. Rowe and Kahn report that people do not adhere to activities that are too difficult. For example, can you put aside five minutes per day to walk? If you commit time to such a minor activity, you will be surprised how far it will lead you and how many benefits will accrue in the long run.

- From the available fitness possibilities, select the one that is in harmony with the natural tendency of your body. The individual uniqueness of your potential is reflected through preference for specific sports and activities. Choose the one that you will most enjoy. Whether you walk, swim, jog, dance, or hike, they all produce similar benefits provided you practice one of them. Consider exercise as a way to peak experiences reflecting your body's chemical reaction for providing it with the oxygen and the movement it needs. It is your organism's way to say "thank you."

- Consult your physician and get his approval for the selected activity.

▪ ▪ ▪

While there is great enthusiasm among practicing seniors regarding the benefits of exercise on health, it is proper to mention a word of caution. Some professionals believe that fitness training has little or no impact on health. Among the conservative physicians is Dr. Henry A. Solomon, respected cardiologist, whose position is expressed in the book *The Exercise Myth*. As the title indicates, the author believes that athletic activities make people feel better, but do not make them healthier.[17] He stresses that "feeling well" does not mean the absence of symptoms. He describes coronary disease as a silent condition that may not produce any noticeable pain or symptomatic discomfort.

To find out whether a beginner is fit to start physical training requires a stress test. But he warns that even a stress test is not an accurate measure of the heart condition because the performance may be affected by temperature, humidity, and the patient's mood, such as anger or depression, and other factors that may bias the test result.

In order to minimize the possibility of cardiac event, Dr. Solomon suggests moderate exercise and stopping at the sign of exhaustion. He advises one to listen to the body and pay attention to what it conveys. It will let the athlete know how far he or she can go. If breathing is more strenuous than usual, the exercise should be discontinued. Even those who are in excellent health should not exceed 75 percent of the heart's maximum rate.[18]

Dr. Solomon's prudent approach will please those seniors who are cautiously optimistic about the value of kinetic impact on an aging body. On the other hand, statistical evidence and numerous studies provide ample evidence that exercise is used in rehabilitation centers as a therapeutic modality. The MacArthur studies indicate that appropriate exercises can prevent frailty and rejuvenate the organism even in very old and regressed individuals.

■ ■ ■

Exercise for youth: Many seniors are asking, "Can exercise reverse the aging process?" Since the definition of aging is elusive, one cannot measure it. What can be measured is the performance before and after exercise, indicating an increase in oxygen intake, improvement of cardiovascular and respiratory capacity, reduction of cholesterol, increase of bone minerals and mass, increase in the flexibility of joints, improvement in bowel functioning, muscle strength, sleep pattern, sensory and intellectual capacity, and much more.

To exercise for youth means to live with an increased awareness of the body's functioning and respond to it by individual exercises as needed.

Mrs. H. was a semiretired journalist who spent a major part of the day sitting at the computer, not noticing that her sedentary lifestyle affected her posture and gait. One day, as she was walking in a department store, she noticed an old women shuffling toward her. After a brief reaction of pity, she realized, to her dismay, that the old woman was herself, reflected in a large mirror. The shock of this confrontation motivated her to enroll in a fitness center where a makeover program was developed for her by a team of trainers. Her weight lifting program consisted of a variety of exercises on machines, pedaling on a bike, and reaching every day a minimum of 5,000 steps. In one year, her posture, gait, and flexibility improved and so did her self-esteem. In her words, it is not only the exercise that made a difference, it is also the awareness of her body that counts. Whenever she now begins to slouch over her computer, she takes a break, rests, and returns to her desk regenerated.

The slogan "no pain, no gain" promoted by some rejuvenation programs contrasts with our approach. Based on an extensive study of existing literature, we summarize those concepts that best suit seniors:

- Physical and spiritual aspects of age reversal are part of the same process.
- Exercising must be safe, enjoyable, even an exhilarating experience.
- To exercise for youth means to enjoy the process while moving toward the goal.
- Practice one or more sports for pleasure.
- To exercise for youth is more than a commitment to selected physical activity. It is a commitment to a purpose that requires us to be young.
- Any and all of the three methods can be practiced as needed: cardiovascular conditioning, power training, and flexibility training.

■ ■ ■

In addition to the established roster of traditional fitness methods, many professionals and gurus are promoting their individual schools of practice offering a wide variety of modern equipment and an expanded range of techniques. From the overwhelming possibilities, we selected one that is responsive to seniors' needs for interaction with others.

Exercising together with a partner may motivate those who do not like to practice alone. If you have a willing spouse, friend, or partner, fitness and self-improvement can become a way of mutual giving through physical contact. The exercise consists of gradual movements that are first self-determined and later structured.

- First, you are sensitized to the presence of another person in your private sphere.
- Verbal communication is not recommended as movement and self-awareness are the body's main messengers.
- As you are moving around your partner, you experience heightened awareness of each other and of sensibility between both of you.
- You are aware of the space between you.
- You do not touch until one of you will initiate a physical contact. It is a message. You experience a reaction that you will express by motion, kinetically, not verbally.
- Slowly a dialogue evolves via movement and touching.
- The contact between partners is monitored by the trainer so that it is not counterproductive.
- After 30 minutes of movements, the body will be more flexible, balanced, and self-aware.

- Repeated exercises progress to varied stretches and other movements that are performed with mutual assistance.[19,20]

■ ■ ■

Millions of Americans live longer and healthier lives than ever before, and thousands of them are becoming younger every year because they are involved in regular exercise. In this extraordinary era of demographic transformation, physical fitness is becoming an agent of positive change. Without the opportunities for manifold forms of physical activities, the capacity of seniors to sustain their independence, health, and individual lifestyles would be considerably diminished. If extended longevity does not keep pace with adequate mobility, aging people could become a mass of physically limited, dependent individuals rather than leaders in a new social order.

In this chapter, presented research results demonstrate that frailty is to a very large extent reversible. Most elderly have the capacity to increase their strength, walking ability, and improve other aspects of functioning. Exercise makes a meaningful difference in overall performance. It is never too late to start to practice if you have the desire, the commitment, and the vision for your future.

11 ▪ ▪ ▪

Vertigo, Dizziness, and Balance

NATAN BAUMAN, ED.D., M.S., ENG., F-AAA

> Honor a physician with the honor due him
> for the uses which ye may have of him;
> for the Lord hath created him.
>
> —Ecclesiasticus 38: 1–2

It is estimated that 90 million Americans will report balance-related symptoms to their physicians at least once in their lifetimes, and 7 million people seek medical assistance every year for treatment of episodic dizziness.[1] These statistics demonstrate that varied forms of vertigo, dizziness, and loss of balance constitute a significant health problem in the United States. By the age of 65, 30 percent of the total population will experience at least one episode of dizziness.[2] Because of the prevalence of these symptoms, one entire chapter is dedicated to the review of this common health problem among seniors, so that they are able to cooperate with their physicians and better understand and cope with these medical problems.

What is dizziness? We all remember the days of our childhoods when we stepped down from the merry-go-round and the world was spinning around us. Then it was fun—now it is an inconvenience and sometimes a threatening affliction. Whether we are affected by a single episode or by reoccurring dizziness symptoms, it is a disorienting, unpleasant experience limiting walking, driving, and other activities. Moreover, as long as we do not know the cause of the episode, we are concerned whether it is a signal of a life-threatening condition or an event not to worry about. Since there are many potential causes for these symptoms, it is a challenge for the physician to determine the origin of the reported discomfort and to succeed at a correct diagnosis and an appropriate treatment.

Mrs. N., 81 years of age, developed persistent dizziness that was not alleviated in spite of adequate rest and a healthy diet. She consulted her physician who examined her and found her in good health. However, the symptoms continued, and Mrs. N. consulted two other doctors. One found her vital signs unremarkable; the other inquired about her medication. Mrs. N. reported that she was using a tranquilizer, prescribed by an out-of-town doctor where she attended the funeral of her sister. The sedative medication was the cause of her dizziness; when it was discontinued and substituted by another brand, her symptoms subsided. She realized that sharing all information with doctors is essential for a fast and accurate diagnosis and treatment.

Because there are varied types of vertigo, the patients should describe their sensations in detail: some are experienced as a dizziness or blackout, some feel as if one is falling down, backward, or sideward or just spinning uncontrollably around. In some cases, additional symptoms are reported, such as nausea, loss of hearing or vision, headache, or tinnitus.

Doctors treating these conditions range from general practioner to neurologist, otolaryngologist, otologist, otoneurologist, to other experts.

The description of the symptomatology of the balance loss and related disorders highlighted in this chapter is intentionally free of medical terminology and of excessive anatomic details, as the purpose here is to empower the readers by a general understanding of symptoms so that they may better understand and identify them should they ever be affected by it. Also, it will help them to discuss treatment alternatives with their physicians from an informed position.

There are three major categories of vertigo and loss of balance based on different etiologies:

- peripheral vestibular disorders;
- presyncope disorders;
- disequilibrium disorders.

We will review their causes, symptoms, and treatment possibilities:

Peripheral vestibular disorders refer to dizziness resulting from a dysfunction in the vestibular system of the inner ear that processes information about equilibrium related to imbalance. This system is part of an extraordinary communication network between several major players, our ears, eyes, feet, and cerebellum, that constantly exchange information with each other regarding our motions: The eyes send messages to the brain about one's position; the organism in the ear, known as the vestibular labyrinths, forwards the messages to the cerebellum via cranial nerves about the position our feet experience, and the brain processes the information. The end result of this complex exchange is our sense of balance. Any disturbance in the communication of this triumvirate may cause vertigo, dizziness, or other symptoms of disequilibrium.

The vestibular labyrinth is an exquisite system consisting of semicircular canals that contain fluids and nerves in the form of fiberlike hairs. Attached to them are calcium crystals called otoconia that pressure the hair by their weight as we move around. The otoconia are in charge of detecting the gravity of the head's motion and conveying information to the brain. It is a common experience that healthy people who are traveling by car or train and read while the vehicle is in motion experience sudden nausea or dizziness. How is this possible? While the eyes are looking at a book that is not moving, the ear labyrinth is sensing the motion of the vehicle and sends a different message to the brain. The discrepancy of information to the brain causes instant dizziness, often accompanied by nausea, that ceases when the reading is discontinued. This example of vestibular disorder demonstrates that balance is maintained as long as the ear, the eyes, and the brain flawlessly cooperate. However, if one of the messengers fails, loss of balance follows.

Vestibular disorders are recognized under several diagnostic categories with slightly different symptoms:

- Benign paroxysmal positional vertigo is a frequently reported condition, caused by the tiny otoconia crystals when they break and roam in the fluid of the vestibular labyrinth. They disrupt the normal flow of balance to the brain until they are repositioned through therapy to a sack called a utricle where they cannot interfere.

   Mr. R. was a vigorous accountant, 78 years of age, who still was practicing in his firm. He ascribed the occasional bout of dizziness to working too hard at his computer. However, a medical examination indicated otherwise: The loss of balance was caused by dislodged otoconia crystals pressing their hairlike receptors in the vestibular labyrinth. Mr. R. was treated by a therapist who used several maneuvers to reposition the crystals to an adjacent sack of utricle where they could not interfere with the balance. Mr. R. practiced some of the maneuvers at home whenever he experienced dizziness.

If any senior wants to reinforce the repositioning exercise at home, we recommend caution, as more harm than benefits can be done by independent treatment.

- Vertigo can also be caused by the inflammation of the inner ear, particularly the labyrinth. This condition, known as neuronitis or labyrinthitis, causes intense vertigo that often lasts for days and may include other symptoms, such as nausea and vomiting. The treatment includes rest in the supine position. The etiology is not known, but it is assumed that it could be caused by a virus as it frequently follows a viral infection in other parts of the body. Appropriate exercise is usually prescribed for this condition, and recovery follows after the intervention.

- Ménière's disease is characterized by sudden episodes of vertigo that usually last several hours and are accompanied by tinnitus and progressive hearing loss. This disorder is caused by intermittent swelling of the labyrinth. The etiology of this condition is unknown. Patients have to be treated by a doctor who will recommend comprehensive audiometry with specialized balance testing and medication to reduce the hearing loss and vertical symptoms. Approximately 80 percent of patients reportedly recover spontaneously within five years,[3] but many of them will continue to experience occasional vertigo after the main condition has been resolved.

- Vestibular migraine is usually experienced by individuals of all ages who are sensitive to motion. It can be triggered by a sudden change of position, riding in a vehicle, or traveling by plane or boat. A migraine may accompany vertigo for several minutes, or the condition may last several days. It is reassuring to know that vertigo is rarely a symptom of a more serious problem and can be treated by doctors rather successfully. However, do not diagnose yourself on the basis of information you read or receive from friends; consult a professional as soon as you can to eliminate misdiagnosis. It is of interest to mention that a headache is sometimes experienced following vertigo or vice versa, and at other times only vertigo occurs; this explains why it is sometimes difficult to distinguish vestibular migraine from other pathologies, for example, a brain tumor.

- Acute peripheral vestibulopathy is characterized by a single acute onset of severe vertigo, nausea, vomiting, and ataxia. This common clinical condition affects people of all ages and lasts from several hours to several days. The therapy consists of bed rest and appropriate medication prescribed by the treating physician.

■ ■ ■

Presyncope disorders include varied types of dizziness that are not related to the vestibular conditions, but rather are caused by an insufficient cardiovascular system. The symptoms are experienced as light-headedness without losing consciousness, nausea, pale skin, blurred vision, and a sense of dizziness[4]

The common diagnostic entities follow:

- Orthostatic hypotension is a common cause of dizziness among seniors. It frequently occurs after quickly standing from a sitting position as a result of inadequate blood flow. When a sudden drop in blood pressure does not meet the brain's minimum requirement, loss of consciousness may follow. The symptom is often preceded by blurred vision or a "blackout" sensation, feeling of weakness, faintness, and occasionally passing out. The balance is restored after one sits or lies down and the systolic blood pressure resumes its normal flow. The underlying cause of the hypotension is either atherosclerosis or arrhythmia.[5]

  Mrs. W., 64 years of age, was dedicated to her family. Before every holiday, she did shopping for her children and many grandchildren, looking for bargains in overcrowded department stores. While standing in a long line at a checkout counter, she suddenly felt weak, dizzy, her vision was blurred, and she was passing out. After sitting for about 30 minutes, her dizziness subsided. She felt much better after she was examined at a walk-in medical center in the neighborhood and was told that her dizziness was not a symptom of a transient ischemic attack, but rather a result of her heart's inability to pump blood vigorously enough to provide the brain with needed oxygenation. The medication prescribed by physicians for the treatment of presyncope includes antihypertensive drugs and elastic venous compression stockings; other medications are considered if they do not interfere with potential congestive heart failure, hepatic cirrhosis, or renal failure.

- Hyperventilation syndrome is another type of presyncope that frequently occurs in individuals of any age who overload their brains with an excessive amount of oxygenation. Such patients are usually anxious, hard-driven individuals who start to hyperventilate when they are excited or are in stressful situations.[6] Hyperventilation is often a sign of underlying anxiety disorder.

A young secretary complained of the occasional feeling of dizziness, blurred vision, and the feeling of passing out after she volunteered to sing in a church choir. The accelerated demand for breathing, together with an ambition to excel, led to overbreathing and hyperventilation. The reassurance of her physician about her condition and its management reduced her anxiety and fainting spells.

- Vasovagal presyncope is very similar to orthostatic hypotension. This episode of light-headedness or dizziness frequently occurs in hot, crowded rooms while the affected person is standing. The symptom is caused by the dilation of arterioles and may occur in healthy people of any age. The best approach to this condition is to avoid places that could lead to an episode of dizziness.

- Cardiac presyncope is another cause of dizziness. It is due to varied heart conditions that might be undiagnosed. Light-headedness or dizziness can be an indication of more serious heart disorders such as coronary ischemia, even if the patient does not report chest pain or other coronary symptoms. I would recommend a thorough examination of the cardiovascular system by a medical professional to avoid any potential risks.

- Micturition presyncope is the usual cause of a ''dizzy spell'' after seniors get up at night to empty their bladders. Sudden vertigo is due to the vasodilatation that may occur at the end of urination, which results from a drop in systolic blood pressure and causes a decrease in cerebral perfusion.[7]

- Hypoglycemia is not a cause of true dizziness, but is mentioned here because patients experience similar symptoms as those reported under presyncope. Hypoglycemia is a metabolic irregularity diagnosed in individuals who are diabetic, prediabetic, or hypersensitive to carbohydrates. They may experience fainting or near fainting spells because their serum glucose dips too low, typically below 17 mg. Medical diagnosis and treatment are warranted.

■ ■ ■

Disequilibrium disorders represent a complex systemic category of symptoms of different etiology from the vestibular and presyncope disorders. This class consists of a range of diseases that interfere with the sensory input of organs, their central integration, and the brain's motor response to it. The disequilibrium is caused by one or more diseases; therefore, it is difficult to diagnose the condition when multiple sensory difficulties are reported.

Seniors experiencing disequilibrium frequently do not feel dizzy or nauseous, but rather report that they are unsteady and insecure when walking and typically tend to hold on to a railing or other people who accompany them.

In systemic disequilibrium, the role of the central nervous system plays a major role as a master coordinator of the sensory input from pertinent organisms, mainly the eyes, the ears, the vestibular system, the feet, and the cerebellum.

Messages from the eyes are the most important factor in informing the brain about one's position, environment, and intended motions. While we walk, we need to see clearly where we are and control the spatial dimensions so that we may move forward safely. It is a common experience that walking at night through a familiar room may cause disoriention and dizziness. Failing vision is a cause of miscommunication with the cerebellum that cannot control our motions and consequently is the cause of many falls. These falls do not have to happen, if timely care is provided when sight begins to show decline.

The distortion of the visual messages may be caused by head trauma, retinopathy, retinoblastoma, degeneration of the macula, glaucoma, and also degenerative conditions such as multiple sclerosis. Those who have had a head trauma in the past must report it to their physicians so that it may be considered in the diagnostic formulation.

The ears are more relevant to our equilibrium than we might imagine. The degenerative diseases of the vestibular system, such as a slowly growing neoplasm (acoustic neuronal) or toxins (aminoglycoside antibiotics), neuropathies as in diabetes mellitus and idiopathic sensory hearing loss, can contribute to the disequilibrium disorders. If we want to test the importance of hearing for balance, we may insert earplugs and walk in a department store or on the streets. The diminishing hearing capacity will distort the ear-cerebellum communication and result in unsteady balance. If the cerebellum does not get the correct messages, it cannot adequately control the motor movements.[8]

The motor movements are determined by the cerebellum and executed by the central nervous system. In the case of a degenerative condition such as Parkinson's disease, neoplasm, or alcohol-related syndrome, a gait disorder will result. Alzheimer's disease, Creutzfeldt-Jacob disease, multiple sclerosis, renal failure, and impairments of the central nervous system may also cause loss of balance. It is a well-known fact to doctors that people suffering from dementia often complain of dizziness.

As is apparent from the aforementioned information, the central nervous system's functioning is vital for sustaining a steady equilibrium.

Mr. E., 71 years of age, recovered from a stroke remarkably well. Prompt rehabilitation and medical care immediately after the event regenerated his facial flexibility and voice, but his left leg was weaker and less sensitive. Mr. E. tended to use his right leg more frequently as the stronger and more sensitive extremity, but complained of reduced postural reflexes when walking. Since the neurological findings indicated the absence of vestibular pathology, the therapy focused on retraining of the communication network between the cerebellum and the nerves in his extremities. One of the exercises that helped considerably to improve his gait was walking in front of a mural mirror and coordinating the visual messages with the physiological experience. This daily 30-minute procedure was so successful that Mr. E. was able to later perform a well-balanced walk with closed eyes.

In order to protect the interplay of activities that our organisms have to produce to maintain balance, we need to make sure that our vision, hearing, proprioception, and the central nervous system are as healthy as possible. Availability of sophisticated medical technology frequently improves vision and hearing to normal levels. We can overcome to a large extent the resistance for self-improvement if we avoid thinking that it is "too late" or we are "too old" and work with determination on controlling our balance and our lives.

The Mayo Clinic Newsletter recommends that patients report the following symptoms to their doctors:

- an unusual type of headache or head injury;
- blurred vision;
- hearing loss;
- speech impairment;
- tinnitus;
- leg or arm weakness;
- loss of consciousness;
- fever higher than 101°F (38.3°C);

- a very stiff neck;
- chest pain or rapid (or slow) heart rate
- falling and difficulty walking,
- numbness and tingling;[9]
- do not forget to inform your doctor(s) about all the medications, vitamins, and supplements you are taking—this can make a difference in the diagnosis.

A number of studies estimate the percentage of falls in seniors 65 years of age and older to be up to 50 percent. Falls are the sixth leading cause of death with a rate of 8.5 percent in 100,000 people between the ages of 65 and 74. The numbers increase to 56.7 percent per 100,000 in those aged 75 and older.[10] The statistics further inform us that 1 percent of falls result in hip fracture, which amount to 200,000 cases per year.[11] In addition, falls cause soft tissue injuries and such fractures as pelvis, humerus, or wrists that are also reported as a contributing factor in nursing home admissions and as an altering factor in the lifestyle of the senior population.

The good news is that you do not need to be part of the above statistics if you maintain your health in good condition and treat symptoms before they become diseases and morbidities. Falls can be to a large extent prevented by increased awareness of what causes them. As indicated in this chapter, the capacity for a stable balance and elimination of dizziness and vertigo can be to a large extent controlled or reduced by early prevention and treatment of diseases of the eyes, ears, vestibular, cardiovascular, and central nervous systems, as well as early communication with the treating physicians. We have great technologies available for improving hearing with hearing aids; visual problems can be corrected surgically or by nonsurgical procedures, and an array of medications exists to treat or delay the progression of degenerative diseases.

The wear and tear of organisms can be alleviated to a large extent by lifestyle and care for general maintenance of which good balance is only a part.

But sometimes, even with the best medical care and self-discipline, an illness, such as a stroke, may happen. Fast action is needed to start rehabilitation. Consequences of stroke frequently include paralysis of legs, sensory loss, and visual dysfunction that affect the balance. While the realization of the damage may first cause hopelessness, we should never give up. A vigorous treatment program may lead to considerable improvements in functioning that is worth the effort. Kirk Douglas, a charismatic Hollywood actor, suffered a stroke that affected not only several organs, but also his vocal cords—the tool of his profession. In spite of a bleak prognosis, he did not give up, but started to train with perseverance and creativity until he was again able to walk and talk. He relied less on the company of people and was often training alone in his pool together with his dog who became his best companion. Douglas appeared in one or more films following his rehabilitation and become a symbol of hope and encouragement to those who are ready to give up: Beyond modern technologies, medicine, and perseverance, it is the spirit over matter that counts.

Pope John Paul II is another example of one living an active lifestyle while affected by a degenerative condition. He suffered from Parkinson's disease for several years, but did not allow the dysfunction to inhibit his apostolic mission and traveled all over the world almost until his death.

Some seniors who experience difficulties with walking due to inadequate balance, dizziness, or vertigo or other related conditions sometimes use their disabilities as an excuse to lean on their spouses or other family members and friends. It is unfortunate that they are giving up on themselves or tend to take it easy and ask for assistance even when they could help themselves with some effort. By doing so, they are increasing day by day their dependency on others, thus diminishing their chances of rehabilitation.

We all make choices that determine our destinies. The fear of loneliness, illness, or death paralyzes us and produces emotional and spiritual inertia, also known as a slow death syndrome. The other choice is the way of courage, faith, and hope that have the power to overcome anxiety and fears and elevate us above entropy.

How to reach the road leading toward mastery of the decay is the theme of the next chapter.

12 ▪ ▪ ▪

The Duality of Being

Matter and Energy are interconvertible.[1]

—Albert Einstein

Albert Einstein's statement that "death means nothing" reflects his conviction that "for believing physicists distinction between present and future is only a stubbornly persisting illusion."[2] Such a perception conveys the quantum vision of life where constant transformation of matter into energy, and vice versa, takes place in the universe; humans cannot escape identical conversion because they are an indivisible part of the field and are subject to its laws.

The cumulative evidence compiled from varied publications points to the fact that death is a notoriously misunderstood event. The fear that it inspires is a mental projection, transmitted from one generation to another during the course of the millennia of human evolution. Unless we separate the myth from the facts, we may be misled into the gloomy illusion that we stop existing when we cease breathing. This generally accepted belief, magnified by the society's emphasis on the physical aspects of the body and the underestimation of energy as ever-lasting, may deprive us from embracing the glorious truth that death is a transformation.

It is estimated that an average body is composed of 7×10^{27} atoms, which is "7" followed by 27 zeros; another way to express this is "seven billion, billion, billion."[3] Even when atoms are split into smaller particles, they do not disappear but change into a new configuration of energy.

The universe is organized with such an inconceivable accuracy and intelligence that no transaction goes unnoticed. Since even microscopic changes in our cells are noticed by the quantum field, it would be absurd to believe that seven times triple billion of atoms that form our bodies could have an end or simply disappear without any trace.

''What happens after we die?'' This is one of the most frequently asked questions in later years. An array of assumptions and theories has been proposed by theologians, philosophers, scientists, and gurus in an attempt to bridge the reality from life on earth to an existence beyond this realm.

The goal of this chapter is to open our minds to the possibilities that death is not an end of life, but rather a transformation of forms and substances. This view will allow us to consider a truth that is more scientific and less anxiety provoking. Alternatives to obsolete beliefs will be presented, which will dispel fears, reduce ignorance of the unknown, and empower us to make informed choices that will determine what will happen to us after we die.

The cynical statements ''when it's over, it's over'' or ''when you are gone, you are gone'' reflect a purely materialistic view. A person is more than a physical body; the organism also consists of spirit and energy that are everlasting. The dualism of body and soul needs to be addressed before we learn from examples of individuals who transcended this life that we also have the potential to achieve our personal immortality.

▧ ▧ ▧

Whenever matter coexists with spirit, there is dualism. The body is mortal and subject to man-made laws that terminate its terrestrial existence through probate courts and the distribution of personal assets to the beneficiaries. The soul is immortal, and, after death, it presumably exists in a disembodied state in the form of energy. But there is more to it: Horace, the Roman poet who lived more than 2,000 years ago, is remembered for his glorious poetry and the statement that became the epitome of immortality: ''Non Omnis Moriar,'' or ''Not all of me will die.''[4] His talent, love, and wisdom continue to live in his verses even though his physical person is no longer present. In reality, death marks the end of only certain functions, while other activities begin. Even though the vital body functions cease, the essence of that person survives in many forms.

Millions of people all over the world incorporate the teachings of the Lord Jesus, Mohammed, Buddha, and other spiritual leaders who lived many thousands of years ago. The moral code established by Moses in the Ten Commandments has outlived its time and serves as a basis for human conduct in all civilized societies today. Socrates did not write a single book, yet his ideas and teachings influence Western civilization in a lasting way. All these men still live in a spiritual form that is part of our everyday lives. We talk to them in distress, try to live according to the standards they set, and follow them as examples of supreme humanity. According to some studies, "the dead do not disappear from the lives of the living. They stay connected and lively communication continues between the two worlds."[5]

But regardless of our relative insignificance, we, too, have the potential to achieve personal immortality if we can rise above our self-interest. A single mother, living in a most perilous neighborhood, had a deep-rooted belief in the liberating effect of education and insisted that her two sons have access to academia. The outcome of maternal concern and dedication to her children resulted in two educated sons. One of them, Benjamin S. Carson Sr., became a great American brain surgeon who did not forget his mother's spiritual heritage. Mindful of the importance of education, he created scholarship funds that rewarded high school students for academic excellence, giving them the opportunity to overcome poverty.[6] The values and beliefs of Carson's mother live in her son and are further transmitted to students who are carriers of Carson's spiritual heritage. A chain reaction, transmitting beliefs in the transforming power of education, may be perpetuated from one generation to another.

Dr. Carson's concern for others is characteristic of generativity, which is an altruistic dedication to establish the succeeding generation not only through financial help, but also by guidance. Our attempt to help those who need us may indefinitely perpetuate our values also. An excerpt from Antoine de Saint-Exupéry's poem "Generation to Generation" poetically expresses the heritage of love that passes from one generation to another:

> If others impart to our children
> our knowledge and ideas,
> they will lose all of us
> that is wordless and full of wonder.

How much profound truth there is in his words:

Let us build memories in our children,
lest they drag out joyless lives,

lest they allow treasures to be lost
because they have not been given the keys.

His memorable words are the essence of life and parental love:

We live, not by things,
but by the meanings of things.
It is needful to transmit passwords
from generation to generation.[7]

Cornell University professor Dr. Urie Bronfenbrenner stated that the future of a nation is determined by the concern that the current generation shows for the well-being and survival of the next one.[8] This statement questions how much we care for the children whom we created, not only during our lifetimes, but also after we are no longer physically present. Our choices determine where our values and priorities are. If we approach the last part of life with the ''après moi le déluge'' (after me the deluge) attitude, we may invalidate many positive and significant accomplishments on which we labored throughout our lives. One's death impacts many people in countless ways, and to leave one's assets without a destination is not a bequest but a burden. Surprisingly, it is estimated that 7 out of 10 American adults die intestate—without a will. What stands in the way of executing a last will to ensure that the individual's property be distributed according to one's wishes?

Some fail to make a will because death makes them feel uncomfortable. Others are too busy, or avoid making a decision about a property, knowing it will be scrutinized by their heirs. Materialistic individuals feel that it does not matter what happens to their assets if they cannot enjoy them. ''Some people refuse to think about practical matters, like their wills, and where they will be buried, because they do not like to think about their death,'' states Billy Graham. ''But some day it will be too late.''[9]

Still, some notable personalities failed to do so: President Abraham Lincoln, one of the leading lawyers of his time, died intestate.

Songwriter George Gershwin died a wealthy man, but did not have a will, as was also the case with Pablo Picasso, Jayne Mansfield, and Rita Hayworth. Billionaire Howard Hughes died intestate because none of his 30 wills was found to be valid. One will was drafted on a napkin. After lengthy trials and payments of hundreds of millions of dollars in unnecessary taxes, his fortune was divided between various distant relatives with whom he hardly had any contact during his life, as stated by Herbert E. Nass, Esq., author of *Wills of the Rich & Famous*.[10]

Intestate estates cost needless court and attorney fees that often consume millions of inheritance dollars when a conflict among beneficiaries arises. It is more than foolish to let the state parcel out a property that was often accumulated by sacrifices.

When we move from one dwelling to another, we take great care of our possessions so that they are moved safely to the new home. Surprisingly, when we move from one state of being to another, we are much less prepared for such a great transition, and too many of us leave our energy, congealed in accounts and other valuables, without assignment.

President John F. Kennedy was a busy man caring for the nation first. Following the moment of his sudden death, it was revealed that his will was signed at the time when he was still a senator and before his children were born.[11] He did not update the will when he became president. Nobody expected that he would be assassinated at the young age of 46. The ancient scriptures tell us to live as if we would be called today, but most of us live as if we are not hearing the voice of destiny.

Conrad N. Hilton, who originated from humble beginnings, never forgot what it meant to be poor. He was a tireless worker and during his lifetime developed a personal philosophy from the observation, study, and contemplation of life. His conclusions led him to the formulation of a code of ethics that he made available not only to his children, but also to those interested in a life of purpose. His manifesto is too long to be quoted in its entirety, but some passages are reflective of the deep religious feeling of this exceptional man. "There is a natural law—a Divine law—that obliges you and me to relieve the suffering, the distressed and the destitute. Charity is a supreme virtue, and the great channel through which the mercy of God is passed on mankind."[12] Hilton also established a charitable organization, the Conrad N. Hilton Foundation, to support varied causes related to health, education, and the protection of children. He was a man who was practicing what he preached.

Besides the symbolic act of transmitting the torch of spiritual heritage to the next generation, it is pertinent to clarify an aspect of material inheritance that is often misunderstood. The astonishing reality that generally goes unnoticed is the extraordinary amount of energy we leave behind: living energy congealed in the monetary form. I discovered the far-reaching significance of money under the following unusual circumstances:

In the mid-1950s, I participated in a project in experimental psychology that brought me to the remote parts of the Ituri Forest in the Central Congo, the territory of Pygmies from the Bambuti tribe. One early morning, an old elephant hunter waited for me at the camp. He was shivering with fear. What could possibly cause such a fright in a man who was known as a fearless hunter of the greatest of pachyderms?

The Bambuti translator explained that the man was left behind by his tribesmen because he was too old to hunt and was unable to provide his own subsistence. He was left to die. Without cooperation of the tribesmen, no man can survive alone for long in the rainforest. The old man asked for a "magical medicine" that would restore his strength.

In the wild, food needed for one day of survival is equivalent to the amount of energy expended on extrication of that food from the environment. Reserves of food in the rainforest are hardly possible as everything decays quickly in the hot, humid climate or is devoured by insects and rodents. As humans became civilized, we lost the connection to the nature from which we originated. The farther we go from the wild, the less we understand the basic interaction between the matter and energy needed for survival.

This episode was a shocking revelation of the "quid pro quo" principle of universal survival—no energy, no survival. I could not return the strength to the old hunter by providing him with a magical pill, but I left cash with the director of the Epulu camp, Jean de Medina, to provide food for the Pygmy after our expedition left. In an environment where compassion was an unknown word, and social programs for the elderly a Utopia, my bank notes were elevated above their commercial value: They represented *my energy,* congealed in the form of money, that saved the old hunter's life.

"All money is congealed energy," stated Joseph Campbell. "The mystery of higher consciousness is expressed in the field of money. How we spend it is a matter of realization of what it represents."[13] If we waste our congealed energy on something that is not needed, enjoyed, or is thrown away, we are nullifying the energy. If we give money for a child's education in order for him or her to learn new skills, we are multiplying energy. If we donate money to a scholarship, we are starting a chain reaction that will perpetuate our congealed energy by empowering many more individuals to transform matter into energy of knowledge. Buying drugs to get "high" brings anyone to a low level of being and turns the energy into nothingness. Actions that do not produce any change are not rewarded by an increase in energy level, but follow the path of entropy and deterioration.

The energy we spent during our lives on living and working is the same energy that is distributed after our deaths through our assets. The congealed form of this energy does not change its value and can have the same power to initiate action and make people think according to our guidelines. Einstein equated mass with stored energy, which, under proper circumstances, can produce energy equivalent to the amount of mass. When you prepare a last will and testament, you do not want your energy to be squandered by your heirs' addictive gambling, unsafe investments, or purposes of which you would not approve. As long as your money or other assets exist, your energy lives in them. Your choices expressed in a will determine whether they will be used for lower or higher purposes.

Benjamin Franklin bequeathed $4,400 in 1785 to the cities of Boston and Philadelphia and placed it in a trust for 200 years. As of 1990, more than $2,000,000 accumulated in interest and in 1990 the trust fund amounted to $5,000,000. It was used to establish a trade school that became the Franklin Institute of Boston.[14]

What is your plan for making a lasting impression on the earth?

"Dying with billions of dollars, and having everybody glad that you are gone, does not define a life of value, or life well-spent," states Dr. Carson. "When I talk about a success—full life, I mean a life that benefits the people around you. One can die penniless, as Mother Teresa, and have an enormous impact on the lives of others."[15]

There are many ways to assign assets to people or organizations that will perpetuate your intentions. Inheritances remitted to the beneficiaries by way of a will can be potentially contested, and your wishes might not be executed as desired. Each will must pass probate, a state procedure that controls the distribution of an estate. Because of excessive delays, complications, and the cost of probate, many seniors prefer to establish trusts that do not pass through the probate, but are remitted directly to the beneficiaries.

Among those known for having established trusts for their loved ones were Elvis Presley, Bing Crosby, John Lennon, Fred Astaire, Walt Disney, and Franklin D. Roosevelt. Humphrey Bogart founded a trust for his wife Lauren Bacall Bogart and also put aside assets in a trust for his two children to assure that they had sufficient funds for their education.

You do not need to be superwealthy to establish security for those you love:

Mr. S., a successful businessman, was concerned that his son, an artist, might become destitute because his earnings were unstable. Rather than to pass his assets through a will, he established a trust to pay his son monthly amounts, thus assuring that he can always live decently. Mrs. R. established a trust for her divorced daughter who was a compulsive spender. The trust instrument allowed payments to the daughter only after she reached the age of 50, not leaving any assets while she could still work and support herself. Mr. C. established a trust for his daughter with Down syndrome so that she may live with a housekeeper at an apartment in the community where she grew up.

But even seniors without any material assets may leave something of value to their heirs. Beside trusts and financial bequests, it is increasingly popular to develop a spiritual legacy for future generations. Everybody has words of wisdom or an experience that could be significant to someone else. Even though our children and grandchildren are known for notoriously rejecting parental advice, their attitude changes later in life as they mature.

What does a spiritual testament say about a person who leaves it? As an example of a well-defined legacy, the full text of John D. Rockefeller Jr.'s manifesto follows:

> I believe in the supreme worth of the individual and his right to life, liberty and the pursuit of happiness. I believe that every right implies a responsibility; every opportunity, an obligation; every possession, a duty.

I believe that the law was made for man and not man for the law; that government is the servant of the people and not their master. I believe in the dignity of labor, whether with head or hand; that the world owes no man a living but that it owes every man an opportunity to make a living. I believe that thrift is essential to well ordered living and that economy is a prime requisite of a sound financial structure, whether in government, business or personal affairs. I believe that truth and justice are fundamental to an enduring social order. I believe in the sacredness of a promise, that a man's word should be as good as his bond; that character—not wealth or power or position—is of supreme worth. I believe that the rendering of useful service is the common duty of mankind and that only in the purifying fire of sacrifice is the dross of selfishness consumed and the greatness of human soul set free. I believe in an all-wise and all-loving God, named by whatever name, and that the individual's highest fulfillment, greatest happiness, and widest usefulness are to be found in living harmony with his will. I believe that love is the greatest thing in the world; that it alone can overcome hate; that right can and will triumph over might.[16]

We do not need to be educated to formulate a spiritual legacy or to bequest an object of symbolic value to our posterity or those we love. Perhaps the most touching aspect of the will of Thomas Jefferson, the third president of the United States, was the gift of his gold-mounted walking staff to his friend and successor, President James Madison. It was "a token of the cordial and affectionate friendship which for nearly a half century has united us in the same principles and pursuits of what we have deemed for the greatest good of our country."[17]

My grandfather, whom I never met, was a promising mayor and attorney general in a small Austrian town when he died at the age of 42 years in the midst of World War I. His considerable wealth was wasted following the collapse of the postwar imperial economy, and years later all that was left of his life was a paperweight from his official desk. I was a teenager when I discovered the paperweight in the attic during World War II. My grandfather's story touched me, so I decided in a youthful vigor that I would finish the race for him. There is a long way from an idea to the execution of a plan. It was only later in life, as an established professional, that I had time to fulfill the original goal.

I commissioned grandfather's life-size portrait, which, inserted in a golden frame, was installed in his former office at the town hall, in the presence of the acting mayor and his staff. The symbolic return of a man to his office, nine decades after his death, was a striking experience. When the local historian started to enumerate grandfather's accomplishments, such as the building of a modern school that still serves its purpose and a local savings bank he co-founded, I realized that death, as a biological event, was superseded by continuation of a life process that transformed his investments of energy into lasting values. His invisible persona still lived in the edifices he realized, and his visible biological continuation carried on his genetic code in me. ''Reality exists independently from our ability to observe it,'' stated Einstein.[18] In this sense, I had the gratifying feeling that grandfather's life circle had been completed: His young family survived and the work he accomplished, in a short lifetime, continued to serve people in the community.

▦ ▦ ▦

When planning an estate, it is essential to remember that a will is not a matter of death but of life. Regardless of the format of the legal instrument or of its material, moral, and spiritual contexts, it is vital that we do not give up on ourselves and accept the responsibility for the continuation of our lives after death. As already mentioned, we survive in many forms and need to instruct those whom we leave behind about our intentions. Preparing a will is an affirmation of the courage to live.

To outlive death through monetary trusts and donations to non-profit organizations is the chosen way of the ''rich and famous.'' In addition to personal bequests, Nelson A. Rockefeller, Malcolm Forbes, President Franklin D. Roosevelt, and many others established foundations for specific purposes, which keep their names and heritages alive. Mr. J. Paul Getty gave a major part of his estate to found The J. Paul Getty Museum in Malibu, California, endowing it with $1 billion. Andy Warhol left a vast part of his assets to The Andy Warhol Foundation for the Visual Arts. President George Washington topped off the secular wills by a bequest of high human value: He ordered that all of his slaves receive freedom at the death of his wife, Martha.

Unlike secular trusts and wills, spiritual legacies are intended to keep alive the individual uniqueness of the departed. Whether it is just an accidentally recorded speech, song, or a prepared message to the family members, a documentary, a family genealogicical tree, photograph albums with names and stories of ancestors, genograms, or paraphernalia, they all shed light on the characteristics of the deceased and revive the continuation between generations.

Einstein's advice to his young son Edward was, "Life is like riding a bicycle; to keep your balance you must keep moving."[19] John J. Astor IV, while helping his expecting wife into the lifeboat during the sinking of the RMS *Titanic,* reportedly said, "Good bye darling, I will see you later."[20] Andy Warhol's contempt for accepted standards personified his attitude about death: "Death means a lot of money, honey."[21] Malcolm S. Forbes directed that his epitaph read "While alive, he lived."[22] Romans of ancient times liked to chisel only one word on their gravestones: "VIXIT"—I lived. Mark Twain, a prankster during his life, once arranged the printing of his obituary in New York while he traveled in Europe. After the notice of his death appeared in the news, he sent from Europe the following cable: "The reports of my death are greatly exaggerated."[23]

The power of the physiological survival cannot be underestimated. Genetic testing can trace the origin of individuals who lived hundreds and thousands of years ago. From generation to generation, people carry physical structures and the genetic codes of their ancestors. Their attributes, programmed by biological factors, include inherited potentialities and talents that may be developed by descendents based on the laws of heredity.

The longevity of our beliefs and values has a survival rate more impressive and lasting than any physiological equivalents. A lasting medium for immortality is the passing and integration of values and beliefs. Children learn from their parents by observing them, and their internal navigational system for making it in life is, to a large extent, a result of internalized values and beliefs. If they grow up in the presence of hatred, violence, and the belief that life is not worth living, they will pass such detrimental ideas onto their children, thus perpetuating the cycle of negative energy. We all have the power to transform a low-level relationship to a positive, high-level energy interaction with others. What a great heritage we can leave to our decendents if we become the personification of the best in us, of love that heals. Death is an act of disappearance only if there is no concern for those we leave behind, for they are defined by our actions during life and beyond.

''We ought, so far as it is in our power, to aspire to immortality, and do all that we can to live in conformity with the highest that is within us; for even in small quantities, its power and preciousness far exceed anything else.''[24] Since Aristotle wrote these words over 2,400 years ago, they still represent a lasting truth. When the precious moments that we spent with our loved ones become integrated into their subconsciousness and memory, Aristotle's word about our immortality will be fulfilled: An experience of love becomes the source of lasting comfort and of the potential to pass it in manifold forms to the next generation.

We cannot defeat entropy and passage of time by fighting it, but rather, by elevating ourselves to a higher human level, above the terrestrial dust of which our bodies are made and transcending life itself. For in the power of love is our salvation.

When Greek philosopher Heraclitus of Ephesus recognized the central role of nature's transformation as part of a changing cosmos, he taught us that life and death, as a process, are also part of the universal change. At the moment of crossing the bridge from here to there, we are not leaving but only experiencing a metamorphosis, which is a part of the universal continuum without an end. The mystical proximity of the ultimate change calls for the connection with love of one's true self that has the power to outgrow the lower pull of biology and reach toward the fusion with the ultimate radiance and bliss.

How can we prepare for the crossing of the bridge?

On the question, what would he do three minutes before death, George B. Shaw reportedly answered that he would learn a new foreign word.

We all create our own vision of the world and the afterlife. After leaving the earthly reality of time and space, labor and pain, we are returning to the quintessence of the celestial womb from which we came. Until then, let us live and love until the last minute.

13 ▪ ▪ ▪

Journey Toward the Light

Behold, I show you a mystery, We shall not all sleep, but we shall all be changed.''[1]

—I Corinthians 15: 51

The final chapter of this book is not about the end of life, but rather about the beginning of new possibilities beyond this place and time. To answer the question, "What is our destiny after we finish the mission down here?" is both simple and multidimensional. Depending on the choices we make, our bodies are transformed into ashes by cremation, into dust by internment, or are preserved by mummification, deep-freezing, or other procedures. But, we are much more than only a physical body. What happens to our souls?

Theologians, philosophers, gurus, and rishis all elaborate different versions of the afterlife; however, in the final analysis their essence is identical: The soul cannot die because it is spirit beyond all matter.

"The Vedic rishis believed that through incarnation the consciousness becomes new even as it uses materials that can never by created or destroyed," stated Chopra in his groundbreaking best seller *Life After Death*. The afterlife is an opportunity to expand life beyond known boundaries.[2]

The Judaic tradition evolved from the pessimistic notion in Job's story that "a person who goes to the grave will never come from it." However, the later literature, in Daniel, considers death as a "sleep" from which "some will awaken to everlasting life...some to everlasting torment."[3]

The position of biblical writers was expressed in the concept that if we are a part of God now, we also will be a part of Him later. Heaven is the unification with God, while hell is the separation from Him.

The Christian concept of resurrection is presented by Apostle Paul in his letter to the Corinthians:

> All flesh is not the same flesh. There are celestial bodies, and bodies terrestrial...So also in the resurrection of the dead it is sown a physical body, it is raised a spiritual body...Now I say, that flesh and blood cannot inherit the kingdom of God.... We shall not sleep, but we shall all be changed. In a moment the dead shall be raised incorruptible and the mortal must put on immortality; then shall be brought to pass the saying that is written: Death is swallowed up in victory. O death, where is thy sting? O grave, where is thy victory?[4]

In Buddhism, the final release from the cycle of reincarnation is the result of extinction of individual passion, hatred, and delusion. Nirvana is the unconditioned state beyond birth and death that is reached after all cravings have been mortified and all karma, which is the cause of rebirth, has been dissolved. "Rebirth does not involve the transfer of substance, but rather is the continuation of a process," states Master Dogen.[5] Tibetan Buddhists and Hindus alike believe that the last thought at the moment of death determines the character of the incarnation.

In Islam, the basic premise of the Qur'an is the idea that after death a person's conduct is judged by Allah. The Book of Deeds, recording the good and bad actions of everyone, is opened and each person will be consigned either to everlasting bliss or everlasting torment.

The Hellenistic concept of immortality influenced the Western thoughts of spiritual survival. In the Athenian democracy, what mattered was the personal immortality achieved through deeds that benefited the community, the *polis*. Pythagoras claimed that individual conduct during life determines the destiny of the soul after death. The succession of rebirth and death could influence transmigration of the soul that leads to eventual liberation through the union with the Divine and Universal Absolute.

Marcus Aurelius saw in death an important test of human conduct, influencing actions toward higher goals, a catalyst stimulating citizens during life toward greater goodness. Socrates, when condemned to death, described the life beyond as a bliss.

According to an exclusive survey of 1,011 AARP members, 50 years of age and older, 80 percent responded that they will go to Heaven after death, 20 percent believed in Hell, and 20 percent believed in reincarnation.[6]

All of the spiritual and religious traditions have one idea in common: They firmly believe in the survival of the soul after death. For a believer, the immortality of the soul is a matter of acceptance of the transcendental without questioning it. For a physicist, it is a matter of a search for the higher truth beyond spirituality that depends on ongoing scientific inquiry. A new understanding of the world and the universe deepens knowledge and reveals unexpected possibilities for humankind.

When a person expires in rural parts of Europe, family members open the window so that the soul may leave. This centuries-old tradition reflects the popular belief that part of the deceased continues to exist beyond the here and now. But what is the destination of the soul after it leaves the body? Where does it go? In what substance and state does it exist?

The dualism of matter and spiritual energy is apparent in the cosmos as well as it is in the body. Besides the spiritual realm, symbolized by invisible God or, depending on cultures, other deities, there is the visible, physical universe made of billions of stars, dark matter, and phenomena that can be observed with high-tech instruments.

On the micro level, space is filled with superstrings, the smallest, indivisible constituents of matter thus far identified. They are some "hundred billion billion times smaller than a single atomic nucleus," states Columbia University physicist Brian Greene.[7] Even with the most powerful atomic smashers, the strings appear only as hardly visible dots. The mass of one's body is made of atoms that consist 99 percent of empty spaces. However, the vacuum is filled with vibrating strings of energy and intelligence that connect us to the universe during our lifetime, but they vibrate even through inanimate matter. "At the ultramicroscopic level, the interaction would be akin to a string symphony, vibrating matter into existence," states Greene.[8]

According to medical opinion, human consciousness can be experienced only in a living body because the awareness of self ends with the death of the brain. However, we are part of the universe that is filled with inconceivable intelligence and awareness. It seems rather logical that, following death, our subatomic particles merge with the field:

Where else would they go? There is no escape from the universe. Einstein's famous equation $E = mc^2$ is a reminder that we cannot disappear because, according to the formula, any transformation of matter into energy, or energy into matter, must be equivalent to the total, before and after the change.[9] Living or dead, we represent a universal factor that is here to stay in one substance or another.

The tantalizing question is whether the vibrating particles of energy survive with some elementary traces of our intelligence or rather merge with the vastness of the universe, much like a drop of water in the ocean.

Astrophysicists describe the universe as a cosmic soup with intensive communication and awareness, keeping itself informed of any change through the interaction of everlasting particles. If the microscopic cellular changes in our bodies are noticed by the field, then such a major event as the body's death is also acknowledged. An extraordinary cosmic communication was discovered by physicist John Bell and his co-workers. In carefully arranged laboratory conditions, they observed that two electrons, which were originally entangled, or knew each other, communicated in spite of huge distances; space did not prevent their interconnectedness. Whatever one electron did, the other did also and simultaneously. "An object over there does care about what you do to another object over here," stated Greene.[10] If we exhale an electron in here, it can be on the other side of the moon in no time. If a spaceship left at the fastest available speed to the Andromeda Galaxy, it would take 3 million years to get there; but, an electron, identified by a detector in New York City, could cause the electron in the Andromeda Galaxy to react instantaneously. What unknown mechanism enforces the communication with such spectacular efficiency? How does the particle in Andromeda know how to react simultaneously? "In the quantum world everything has both particles and a wavelike attribute that communicate," states Greene.[11] Photons can traverse the universe while we are taking a step. Does it mean that pairs of particles that were part of our bodies could manifest similar intercommunication? Even if such speculations seem to be farfetched, we cannot refute them totally, because the dreams and hypotheses of today may be the reality of tomorrow.

Quantum exploration of expanded life beyond this universe continues on the premises of analogies: As is the microcosm, so is the macrocosm. It was mentioned previously that humans are born from an ovum, so small that it cannot be seen with a bare eye. Likewise, the universe came into being from a particle smaller than an atom at the moment of the Big Bang. By escalating the continuum of possibilities, is there something bigger than cosmos?

Our universe is estimated to contain a hundred billion galaxies, each filled with a hundred billion stars. In the center of galaxies are black holes known as the shredding places of collapsed stars and interstellar debris. For example, the power of black holes in the Milky Way Galaxy is estimated to be equivalent to 20 solar masses with a diameter of 8 million kilometers. According to Gleiser, the schematic model of black holes indicates that their gravitational force is so enormous that nothing can escape their pull. Even light, speeding at 300,000 kilometers per second, is sucked into the black holes, a pit of no return.

Einstein was intrigued by the phenomenon of black holes at a time when it was not yet confirmed that the universe was expanding. Together with his colleague Nathan Rosen, they pondered the idea of spatial dimensions beyond the one we can see. In his paper "Cosmological Considerations on the General Theory of Relativity," he tried to find quantum reasoning for the black holes. According to his and other studies, it was believed that the black holes connect two spatial locations in the universe. "What the black holes take in, the 'white' hole spits out on the other side," reiterates Gleiser.[12] The Einstein-Rosen bridge was a mathematical formula connecting the center of the black hole with a mirror universe on the "other side" of the space-time.

The question "What is on the other side of this universe?" is answered by exploration of the cosmos by such NASA satellites as Chandra and Swift. They revealed, in pictures, the details of new formations of black holes resulting from giant explosions of massive stars unable to carry their own weight. The gases and mass from the explosions are sucked into the black hole "and disappears from the universe," states Robert Naeye from the NASA Goddard Space Flight Center.[13] To bring evidence that there is another universe is hindered by the fact that the center of the black holes cannot be explored; it is a point of infinite curvature where gravity is estimated to be so powerful that all matter would be crushed to its most fundamental constituents.

The courage of astrophysicists to explore unknown destinations reminds us of the European navigators in antiquity, who, looking over the Atlantic Ocean toward the West, believed that there was an end to the world. Instead, there was a new continent that is now our home. When modern astrophysicists inform us about the possibility of cosmoids and "multiverses" on the other side of our universe, we can only wait and see whether some places "over there" will be the next home of our descendants, de facto or in spirit.

▨ ▨ ▨

Life and the future beyond it are defined by our beliefs. The anticipation of possibilities that may exist on the other side of the bridge are influenced by religious beliefs, scientific convictions, and individual desire. While rational thought processes are controlled by the brain, unconsciousness is connected to the field, which is beyond our control. According to Dr. Sigmund Freud, we can get a glimpse into the inaccessible part of the psyche through our dreams. Based on a series of death dreams that were analyzed by Jungian psychotherapist Marie-Louise von Franz, we were informed that individuals who were facing death did not dream about preparation for an end, but rather a profound transformation and continuation of the life process. Many of the dreams revealed a journey through a dark passage toward light at the end of a tunnel.[14]

The notion that life continues in some form after death is one of the oldest concepts held by mankind. The latter dream analogy reminds us of the difficult human passage through the birth canal with light and life on the end of it. Does it suggest, in transcendental terms, that the soul, following the darkness of death, also continues its existence toward light and new life?

The concept that the universe is recycling its matter is a generally accepted idea by astrophysicists. New stellar bodies are born from the dust, hydrogen, helium, carbon, and oxygen of dying stars, thus suggesting a precedent for the same cycle of birth, death, and rebirth on microcosmic levels.

"We stop fearing death when we stop considering it as an end of life and begin to see it as a continuation of events without time and space," states David Hawkins, author of *The Eye of the I*.[15] We existed as energy before we came to the world, and we continue to exist beyond our existence down here not only on a higher everlasting level, but also through the living part of our bodies that we are leaving behind in our descendents.

When we accept life as a continuation of events that evolve indefinitely in one form or another, death becomes only one of many transformations of our dual existence. Matter becomes energy and vice versa, whereas the soul is immortal and not subject to death. It is here to stay in the presence of God in an infinite, everlasting state.

Mankind's never-ending quest to penetrate the mystery of the afterlife is occasionally rewarded by rare moments of enlightenment. Whether it be through close personal relationships or other occurrences that Einstein described as "rapture" and Maslow as "peak experiences," we seem to be elevated to a state of profound bliss and timelessness. Campbell referred to such a moment as "eternity," a state beyond time. "Eternity...is that dimension of here and now that all thinking in temporal terms cuts off. You can have it right here in experiencing earthly relationships," he said.[16] It is timeless rapture elevating us above the material self.

The most magnificent state of transformed being cannot be described because it transcends words and thoughts. The answer to human desire to meet the divine, as far as we can imagine it, might be the infinite state of eternity. To be filled with the radiance of God's beatific presence could indeed be eternal heaven.

Epilogue

Many decades ago, I studied group therapy under the influential professor Dr. William J. Schwartz, teaching at Columbia University. My first field group consisted of depressed, dysfunctional parents. On the day of the first session, a snowstorm took place and only one parent arrived. I called Dr. Schwartz to consult whether I could cancel the meeting.

"Absolutely not," said the great professor. "You save one person—and you saved humanity."

There is an analogy between my first group session and the spirit in which this book was written. If readers find at least one idea, sentence, or concept that enriches their lives with new insight or is beneficial in any way, then this book was not written in vain.

Olga B. Spencer, Ph.D.

Notes

CHAPTER 1: THE FOUNTAIN OF YOUTH

1. Michael Matousek, "Big Idea," *AARP Bulletin* (July–August 2007): 36.

2. Daniel Goleman, *Social Intelligence: The New Science of Human Relationships* (New York: Bantam Books, 2007), 157.

3. Robert N. Butler, M.D., *Why Survive? Being Old in America* (New York: Harper & Row, 1975), 364.

4. Bernie S. Siegel, M.D., *Love, Medicine & Miracles* (New York: Harper & Row, 1986), 66.

5. Ibid.

6. Karen Horney, *Neurosis and Human Growth* (New York: W.W. Norton and Company, 1950).

7. "Old Testament, The Book of Psalms," in *The Dartmouth Bible,* Sentry ed. (Boston: Houghton Mifflin, 1965), 42.

8. Joseph Campbell, *The Power of Myth* (New York: Doubleday, 1988), 285.

9. *Runner's World* 38, no. 4 (April 2003), retrieved on February 15, 2008, from Academic OneFile database; *Runner's World* 38, no. 1, January 2003, retrieved on February 15, 2008, from Academic OneFile database.

10. Butler, *Why Survive?,* 366.

11. Robert N. Butler, M.D., "Stepping Into the Future," AARP Regional Conference on Aging, Westport, CT.

12. Butler, *Why Survive?,* 367.

13. Ibid., 357.

14. D. Berry, et al, "Move for Longevity," *Consumer Reports on Health,* April 2, 2007, 4.

15. Michael F. Roizen, M.D., *The RealAge Makeover* (New York: Harper Collins, 2004), 304.

16. Gary Small, M.D., *The Longevity Bible: 8 Essential Strategies for Keeping Your Mind Sharp and Your Body Young* (New York: Hyperion, 2006), 140.

17. J. Nesselroade, K. Schaie, and P.B. Baltes, "Improvement of Crystallized Intelligence," *Journal of Gerontology* 27: 222–231.

18. http://thinkexist.com/quotation/it_takes_a_long_time_to_grow_young/341105.html.

19. Ellen J. Langer, *Mindfulness* (Reading, MA: Addison-Wesley, 1989).

20. Ibid., 82–84.

21. Daniel Goleman, *Emotional Intelligence: Why It Can Matter More Than IQ* (New York: Bantam Books, 1995), 167–69.

22. Ibid., 166–68.

23. T.S. Eliot, *The Confidential Club* (New York: Harcourt, Brace and Compass, 1954), 43.

CHAPTER 2: THE FOURTH AGE

1. Caleb E. Finch, "Longevity, Senescence and Genetics of Aging," *Science* (1997): 278–407; James F. Fries and Laurence M. Crapo, *Vitality and Aging: Implications of the Rectangular Curve* (San Francisco: W.H. Freedman Company, 1991), 108–9, 111, 113, 121.

2. S. Jay Olshansky, et al, "More for Longevity," *Consumer Report on Health* 19, no. 4 (April 2007).

3. Roizen, *The RealAge Makeover*, 436.

4. Itzhak Aharon, et al, "Beautiful Faces Have Variable Research Value: MRS and Behavioral Endurance," *Neuron* 32 (2001): 535–51.

5. Small, *The Longevity Bible*, 104.

6. Self-hypnosis is a technique aiming at relaxation, stress reduction, improved concentration, and sleep induction. It can be acquired with professional help and practice.

7. John W. Rowe, M.D., and Robert L. Kahn, Ph.D., *Successful Aging* (New York: Dell Trade, 1998), 45–46.

8. Phyllis A. Balch, CNC, and James R. Balch, M.D., *Prescription for Dietary Wellness: Using Foods to Heal* (New York: Avery, 1992), 183.

CHAPTER 3: THE PURPOSE

1. Emily Dickinson, *The Poems of Emily Dickinson* (Cambridge, MA: Belknap Press of Harvard University Press, 1998), 433.

2. Butler, *Why Survive?*

3. Horace B. Deets, "The Longevity Bonus," *AARP Bulletin* (2000): 28.

4. U.S. Census Bureau Web site, "300 Million and Counting," *AARP Bulletin* (October 2006): 3.

5. Olga B. Spencer, 2000, Survey of 121 seniors, Questionnaire #12-13, AARP Westport-Weston, CT.

6. Excerpt from a conversation with a baby boomer, 2001.

7. Samuel Brandon, "Time and the Destiny of Man," in *The Voices of Time: A Cooperative Survey of Man's Views of Time as Expressed by the Sciences and by the Humanities,* ed. J.T. Fraser (London: Penguin Press, 1968), 157.

8. Campbell, *The Power of Myth,* 186–87.

9. Plato, "Euthydemus," in *Works of Plato,* trans. B. Jowett (New York: Tudor, 1892), 234.

10. Carl R. Rogers and Ruth C. Sanford, "Basic Concepts of Self-Actualizing Tendency," in *Textbook of Psychiatry,* 4th ed., eds. H.E. Kaplan and B.J. Sadock (Baltimore: Williams & Wilkins, 1985), 1382.

11. Ibid.

12. George T. Ainsworth-Land, *Grow or Die: The Unifying Principle of Transformation* (New York: Random House, 1973).

13. Abraham H. Maslow, *The Farther Reaches of Human Nature* (New York: Penguin Press, 1972), 26–27.

14. T.D.A. Lingo, "Dormancy of the Human Brain, Research Report," Dormant Brain Research and Development Laboratory, based on the lecture of Sir John Eccles, University of Colorado, Boulder, July 31, 1974: 1.

15. What is consciousness? A suitable analogy of conscious and unconscious living is our breathing. Most of us hardly ever consciously pay attention to it. Improper breathing can lead to a reduced amount of oxygen and consequent elimination of carbon dioxide from the system. Other functions that depend on breathing may lead to a series of health difficulties. Conscious breathing means to pay attention to the act of breathing at least once a day. Deep breathing oxygenates organisms, reduces stress, and enhances energy. Conscious and unconscious breathing may be extended to any other experience or function of our living.

16. Motoko Rich, "Successful at 96, Writer Has More to Say," *New York Times,* April 7, 2007, B7, 13.

17. Ibid.

18. Ibid.

19. Rowe and Kahn, *Successful Aging,* 47, 168–69.

20. J.A. Wheeler, K.M. Gorey, and B. Greenblatt, "The Beneficial Effect on Older Volunteers on the People They Serve: A Meta-Analysis." *International Journal on Aging and Human Development* (1998): 47, 69.

21. Siegel, *Love, Medicine & Miracles*, 66.

22. Matthew, "Combined Gospels," in *The Dartmouth Bible*, Sentry ed. (Boston: Houghton Mifflin, 1965), 894.

23. Ibid., 894.

24. Victor E. Frankl, *Man's Search for Meaning* (Boston: Beacon, 2006), iii, 138, 140–1.

25. Ibid., iii, 138, 140–1.

26. Ibid., 41.

CHAPTER 4: THE FOUNTAIN OF ENERGY

1. "Motivational and Success Quotes," Millionaire Opportunities, http://www.millionaire-opportunities.com/motivational-and-success-quotes.html.

2. "The Health You Deserve," *Newsletter*, 15 (July 2001), http://www.thewolfeclinic.com/newsletter/newsletter0107.html.

3. "The definition of density is the total energy divided by the volume that contains it." Quoted in Marcelo Gleiser, *The Prophet and the Astronomer* (New York: W.W. Norton & Co., 2002), 183.

4. Gleiser, *The Prophet and the Astronomer*, 179–80.

5. Ibid., 55.

6. Ibid., 228. Two independent groups of astronomers in 1998 discovered that the universe is expanding faster than in the past. They were the Harvard-Smithsonian Center for Astrophysics in Cambridge, Massachusetts, and the Lawrence Berkeley National Laboratory in Berkeley, California.

7. Gleiser, *The Prophet and the Astronomer*, 222–23.

8. Ibid., 228.

9. Brian Greene, *The Fabric of Cosmos* (New York: Alfred A. Knopf, 2004), 432.

10. Frankl, *Man's Search for Meaning*, 20–36.

11. Gleiser, *The Prophet and the Astronomer*, 131–32.

12. Campbell, *The Power of Myth*, 18.

13. Ignacio Martinez and Juan Luis Arsuaga, *Green Fire* (New York: Thunder's Mouth Press, 2003), 14.

14. Horney, *Neurosis and Human Growth*.

15. Deepak Chopra, M.D., *Ageless Body, Timeless Mind* (New York: Three Rivers Press, 1993), 5.

16. John C. Pierrakos, *Core Energetics: Developing the Capacity to Love and Heal* (Mendocino, CA: Life Rhythms Publications, 1987).

17. Dimitri de Berea, 1966, excerpt from *Memoires*, 1990, from the private collection of Olga B. Spencer.

18. Joan LaMontagne, personal letter to the author, September 7, 2007.

19. Maslow, *The Farther Reaches of Human Nature*, 5, 42.

20. Gleiser, *The Prophet and the Astronomer*, 235.

CHAPTER 5: CHANGING FACE OF LOVE AND SENSUALITY

1. Virgil, "Eglogues," in *Petite Larousse*, 4th ed. (Paris: Librarie Larousse, 1962), 10.

2. William H. Masters, M.D., and Virginia E. Johnson, *Human Sexual Response* (Philadelphia: Lippincott Williams & Wilkins, 1966).

3. Rowe and Kahn, *Successful Aging*, 32.

4. Campbell, *The Power of Myth*, 238.

5. John Bowlby, *Attachment and Loss* (New York: Basic Books, 1969).

6. Mark Matousek, "Writing to Live," *AARP Magazine*, April–March 2007, 25–26.

7. Ibid.

8. Rowe and Kahn, *Successful Aging*.

9. Richard Schulz and Timothy A. Salthouse, *Adult Development and Aging: Myths and Emerging Realities* (Upper Saddle River: Prentice Hall, 1993), 252.

10. Ewald W. Busse and George L. Maddox, *The Duke Longitudinal Studies of Normal Aging, 1955–1980: Overview of History, Design and Findings* (New York: Springer Publishing Company, 1985), 226.

11. John C. Pierrakos, *Eros, Love & Sexuality: The Forces That Unify Man and Woman* (Mendocino, CA: LifeRhythm, 2001).

12. Helene E. Fisher, *Anatomy of Love: The Natural History of Monogamy, Adultery and Divorce* (New York: W.W. Norton, 1992), 56.

13. Ibid., 214–15.

14. Phillip C. McGraw, Ph.D., *Relationship Rescue: A Seven-Step Strategy for Reconnecting with Your Partner* (New York: Hyperion, 2001).

15. Aaron T. Beck, *Love Is Never Enough: How Couples Can Overcome Misunderstandings, Resolve Conflicts, and Solve Relationship Problems through Cognitive Therapy* (New York: Harper & Row, 1988).

16. James L. and Nora H. Oshman, *Science Measures the Human Energy Field* (Southfield, MI: International Center for Reiki Training, 2007), 1–7.

17. Diane W. Wardell and Kathryn F. Weymouth, "Review of Studies of Healing Touch," *Journal of Nursing Scholarship*, (2004): 147.

18. Christiane Northrup, M.D., *The Wisdom of Menopause: Creating Physical and Emotional Health and Healing During the Change* (New York: Bantam Books, 2006), 371–74.

19. Ellen K. Torronto, "The Human Touch," *Psychoanalytic Psychotherapy* 18, no. 1 (2001): 37.

20. C. Gehlhaart and P. Dail, "Effectiveness of Healing Touch on Elderly Residents of Long-Term Core Facility on Reducing Pain and Anxiety," *Healing Touch Newsletter* (2000): 3, 8.

CHAPTER 6: THE CREATIVE PROCESS OF LIFE

1. Generativity is a concept developed by E.H. Ericson. It is a power behind various forms of altruistic deeds and caring for the benefit of the succeeding generation and its successful establishment.

2. Martinez and Arsuaga, *Green Fire,* 393–94.

3. Don McLeod, "Matilda Riley's Revolution" (Washington, DC: Research Forum of AARP, 1995), 12.

4. Jonah 1:3 (KJV).

5. David R. Hawkins, M.D., Ph.D., *Power vs. Force: The Hidden Determinants of Human Behavior* (Carlsbad, CA: Hay House, 2002), 282–83.

6. Wayne W. Dyer, *Inspiration: Your Ultimate Calling* (Carlsbad, CA: Hay House, 2006), 17–18.

7. The human ovum weighs only 0.0015 milligrams. Biologist J. Miller calculated that the world's population in the ovum state could be condensed into a one-gallon container. In S.L. Miller, "The Heritage of Copernicus," *The First Laboratory Synthesis of Organic Compounds under Primitive Earth Conditions* (Cambridge, MA: MIT Press, 1974): 228–42.

8. Martinez and Arsuaga, *Green Fire,* 51–54.

9. Alice Calaprice, *Quotable Einstein* (Princeton, NJ: Princeton University Press, 1996), 223.

10. Walter Isaacson, *Einstein* (New York: Simon and Schuster, 2007), 549.

11. Dyer, *Inspiration,* 3.

12. Campbell, *The Power of Myth,* 5.

13. Maslow, *Farther Reaches,* 42.

14. Ibid.

15. Anthony Storr, *The Essential Jung* (Princeton, NJ: Princeton University Press, 1983), 24.

16. Gleiser, *The Prophet and the Astronomer,* 200.

17. Maslow, *Farther Reaches.*

18. Ibid., 32, 171.

CHAPTER 7: EATING TO LIVE STRONGER, LIVE LONGER

1. U.S. Food and Drug Administration, "Center for Food Safety and Applied Nutrition. Dietary Supplements," Warnings and Safety Information. www.cfsan.fda.gov/~dms/supplmnt.html.

2. Northwestern University, "Northwestern Nutrition Fact Sheet: Vitamin C," www.feinberg.northwestern.edu/nutrition/factsheets/vitamin-c.html.

3. B.A. Messina, "Herbal Supplements: Facts and Myths—Talking to Your Patients about Herbal Supplements," *Journal of PeriAnesthesia Nursing* 21, no. 4 (2006): 268–78.

4. Dietary Guidelines for Americans 2005, www.health.gov/dietaryguidelines; DASH Eating Plan 2006; www.nhlbi.nih.gov.

5. Martalena br Purba, et al., "Skin Wrinkling: Can Food Make a Difference?" *Journal of the American College of Nutrition* 20, no. 1 (2001): 71–80.

6. W. Köpcke and J. Krutmann, "Protection from Sunburn with β-Carotene—A Meta-Analysis," *Photochemistry and Photobiology* 84, no. 2 (2007): 284–88, doi:10.1111/j.1751-1097.2007.00253.x.

7. Purba et al., *Journal of the American College of Nutrition*, p. 98.

8. R. Ricciarelli, et al., "Age-Dependent Increase of Collagenase Expression Can Be Reduced by Alpha-Tocopherol via Protein Kinase C Inhibition," *Free Radical Biology & Medicine* 27 (1999): 729–37.

9. H. Wei, et al., "Isoflavone Genistein: Photoproctection and Clinical Implications in Dermatology," *The Journal of Nutrition* 133 (2003): 3811S–19S.

10. U.S. Department of Agriculture, Agricultural Research Service. 2007. USDA–Iowa State University Database on the Isoflavone Content of Foods, Release 1.4—2007. Nutrient Data Laboratory Web site: http://www .ars.usda.gov/nutrientdata.

11. P.C. Calder, "N-3 Polyunsaturated Fatty Acids, Inflammation, and Inflammatory Diseases," *American Journal of Clinical Nutrition* 83 (2006): 1505S–95S.

12. "Third Report of the National Cholesterol Education Program (NCEP) Expert Panel on Detection, Evaluation, and Treatment of High Blood Cholesterol in Adults (Adult Treatment Panel III)," National Institutes of Health Publication No. 02-5215, September 2002.

13. F.B. Hu, et al., "Fish and Omega-3 Fatty Acid Intake and Risk of Coronary Heart Disease in Women," *Journal of the American Medical Association* 287 (2002): 1815–21.

14. M.C. Morris, et al., "Fish Consumption and Cardiovascular Disease in Physicians' Health Study: A Prospective Study," *American Journal of Epidemiology* 142 (1995): 166–75.

15. J.L. Breslow, "N-3 Fatty Acids and Cardiovascular Disease," *American Journal of Clinical Nutrition* 83 (2006): 1477S–82S.

16. S.K. Gebauer, et al., "N-3 Fatty Acid Dietary Recommendations and Food Sources to Achieve Essentiality and Cardiovascular Benefits," *American Journal of Clinical Nutrition* 83 (2006): 1526S–35S.

17. National Institutes of Health Publication, No. 02-5215, September 2002, v–14.

18. American Heart Association and American Stroke Association. Heart Disease and Stroke Statistics—2006 Update.

19. "The Seventh Report of the Joint National Committee on Prevention, Detection, Evaluation, and Treatment of High Blood Pressure (JNC 7)," NIH Publication No. 04-5230, August 2004.

20. F.M. Sacks, et al., "Effects on Blood Pressure of Reduced Dietary Sodium and the Dietary Approaches to Stop Hypertension (DASH) Diet," *New England Journal of Medicine* 344 (2001): 3–10.

21. American Diabetes Association, "Standards of Medical Care in Diabetes—2008," *Diabetes Care* 31, no. 1 (2008): S12–S54.

22. E.J. Johnson and E.J. Schaefer, "Potential Role of Dietary n-3 Fatty Acids in the Prevention of Dementia and Macular Degeneration," *American Journal of Clinical Nutrition* 83 (2006): 1494S–98S.

23. P.R. Trumbo and K.C. Ellwood, "Lutein and Zeaxanthin Intakes and Risk of Age-Related Macular Degeneration and Cataracts: An Evaluation Using the Food and Drug Administration's Evidence-Based Review System for Health Claims," *American Journal of Clinical Nutrition* 84 (2006): 971–74.

24. C.J. Chiu, et al., "Dietary Glycemic Index and Carbohydrate in Relation to Early Age-Related Macular Degeneration," *American Journal of Clinical Nutrition* 83 (2006): 880–86.

25. J.M. Seddon, et al., "Progression of Age-Related Macular Degeneration. Association with Dietary Fat, Transunsaturated Fat, Nuts, and Fish Intake," *Archives of Ophthalmology* 121 (2003): 1728–37.

26. R. Van Leeuwen, et al., "Dietary Intake of Antioxidants and Risk of Age-Related Macular Degeneration," *Journal of the American Medical Association* 294 (2005): 3101–07.

27. M.C. Morris, et al., "Association of Vegetable and Fruit Consumption with Age-Related Cognitive Change," *Neurology* 67 (2006), 1370–76.

28. Johnson and Schaefer, *American Journal of Clinical Nutrition,* p. 14955.

29. M. Garcia-Alloza, et al., "Curcumin Labels Amyloid Pathology in vivo, Disrupts Existing Plaques, and Partially Restores Distorted Neurites in an Alzheimer Mouse Model," *Journal of Neurochemistry* 102 (2007): 1095–1104.

30. M.P. Mattson, et al., "Suppression of Brain Aging and Neurodegenerative Disorders by Dietary Restriction and Environmental Enrichment: Molecular Mechanisms," *Mechanisms of Ageing and Development* 122 (2001): 757–78.

31. Calder, *American Journal of Clinical Nutrition,* p. 1511S.

32. Joint FAO/WHO Working Group Report on Drafting Guidelines for the Evaluation of Probiotics in Food. London, Ontario, Canada, April 30–May 1, 2002.

33. National Center for Complementary and Alternative Medicine. National Institutes of Health. An Introduction to Probiotics. http://nccam .nih.gov/health/probiotics/index.htm.

34. Calder, *American Journal of Clinical Nutrition*, p. 15125.

35. A.P. Somopoulos, "The Mediterranean Diets: What Is So Special about the Diet of Greece? The Scientific Evidence," *Journal of Nutrition* 131 (2001): 3065S–73S.

36. U.S. Department of Agriculture, Agricultural Research Service. Nutrient Data Laboratory Web site: http://www.ars.usda.gov/nutrientdata.

37. Ibid., 3065S–73S.

38. A. Trichopoulou, et al., "Modified Mediterranean Diet and Survival: EPIC-Elderly Prospective Cohort Study," *British Medical Journal* 330 (2005): 991–98.

39. P.N. Singh, et al., "Does Low Meat Consumption Increase Life Expectancy in Humans?" *American Journal of Clinical Nutrition* 78(suppl) (2003): 526S–32S.

40. L.K. Heilbronn, et al., "Effect of 6-Month Calorie Restriction on Biomarkers of Longevity, Metabolic Adaptation, and Oxidative Stress in Overweight Individuals: A Randomized Controlled Trial," *Journal of the American Medical Association* 295 (2006): 1539–48.

CHAPTER 10: FITNESS AT 50 AND BEYOND

1. Roy J. Shephard, *Aging, Physical Activity, and Health* (Toronto: University of Toronto Kinetics, 1997), 28.

2. Ibid..

3. Herbert A. DeVries, with Dianne Hales, *Fitness after 50* (New York: Charles Scribner's Sons, 1982), 22.

4. Shephard, *Aging, Physical Activity, and Health*, 27.

5. Ibid., 271.

6. Ibid., 27.

7. Robert N. Butler, *Stepping into the Future* (Westport, CT: AARP Regional Conference on Aging, 2004).

8. Roy J. Shephard, *Aging, Physical Activity, and Health*, 5, 50.

9. Ibid., 19.

10. James L. Anders and Martin Cohan, *The Westpoint Fitness and Diet* (New York: Rowson Associates, Inc., 1977), 13.

11. Ibid., 11.

12. Olga B. Spencer, "AARP Survey of Aging, Questions 10 and 33, Westport, Connecticut, 1999–2000.

13. Small, *The Longevity Bible*, 109, 145.

14. Rowe and Kahn, *Successful Aging,* 106.

15. Ibid., 106.

16. Ibid., 99.

17. Henry A. Salomon, M.D., *The Exercise Myth* (San Diego, CA: Harcourt, Brace, Jovanovich Publishers, 1984), 12, 15, 21.

18. Ibid., 23.

19. Jeff Donahue and Nancy D. Aquilon, *One-to-One* (New York: Simon & Schuster, 1984).

20. Kelly McEvenue, *The Actor and the Alexander Technique* (New York: Macmillan, 2001), 57, 79.

CHAPTER 11: VERTIGO, DIZZINESS, AND BALANCE

1. Natan Bauman, "Balance Disorders and Falls in the Aged," presentation for the AARP chapter, Westport, Connecticut, 2008, p. 1.

2. Ibid., p. 1.

3. Judd Jensen, "Vertigo and Dizziness," in *Neurology for the Non-Neurologist,* ed. William J. Weiner and Christopher G. Goetz (New York: Random House, 1999), 170, 173, 174.

4. MayoClinic.com, July 29, 2008, http:/www.mayoclinic.com/health/dizziness/DS00435, pp. 1–2.

5. Jensen, "Vertigo and Dizziness," 176.

6. Ibid., 176–77.

7. Ibid., 178.

8. Ibid., 179.

9. MayoClinic.com, 2.

10. National Safety Council, "Accident Facts," 1988.

11. S.P. Baker and A. Harvey, "Fall Injuries in the Elderly," *Clinics in Geriatric Medicine* 1 (1985): 501–8.

CHAPTER 12: THE DUALITY OF BEING

1. Gleiser, *The Prophet and the Astronomer,* 203.

2. Freeman Dyson, *Disturbing the Universe* (New York: Harper and Row, 1979), 193.

3. Brian Kross, "How Many Atoms Are in the Human Body?", ed. Steve Gagnon (Newpoert News, VA: Jefferson Lab Science Education, 2007), http://education.jlab.org/gov/mathatom_04.html/, p. 1 (accessed October 30, 2007).

4. Q.H.F. Horace, "Odes III, 30:6," in *Petite Larousse,* 4th ed. (Paris: Librarie Larousse, 1962), x.

5. Sandra Beatman, "Communication with the Dead: An Ongoing Experience as Expressed in Arts, Literature and Songs," in *In Between Life and Death,* ed. R.J. Kastenbaum (New York: Springer, 1979), 124–55.

6. Melissa Gotthardt, "Memory Makers," *AARP Magazine,* September–October 2002, 72–74.

7. Antoine de Saint-Exupéry, "Generation to Generation," http://www.poemhunter.com/poem/generation-to-generation/.

8. Urie Bronfenbrenner, interview by the author, The Institute for Single Parent Family, Cornell University, July 1977.

9. Janet Kinosian, "Pilgrim's Progress," *AARP Magazine,* November–December 2007, 26.

10. Herbert E. Nass, Esq., *Wills of the Rich & Famous* (New York: Warner Books, 1991), 268–69.

11. Ibid., 6.

12. Ibid., 248–49.

13. Campbell, *The Power of Myth,* 18–19.

14. John C. Bogle, "Capitalism, Entrepreneurship, and Investing—The 18th Century vs. the 21st Century," The Vanguard Group, 2006, 5–6, http://www.johncbogle.com/speeches/JCB_GPVG0106.pdf.

15. Gotthardt, "Memory Makers," 72–74.

16. John D. Rockefeller, "I Believe," a commercial pamphlet without a date or source.

17. Nass, *Wills of the Rich & Famous,* 136.

18. Isaacson, *Einstein,* 461.

19. Ibid., ix.

20. Nass, *Wills of the Rich & Famous,* 227.

21. Ibid., 210.

22. Ibid., 262.

23. Ibid., 155.

24. Dyer, *Inspiration,* 123.

CHAPTER 13: JOURNEY TOWARD THE LIGHT

1. Saint Paul, "Epistle to Corinthians," in *The Dartmouth Bible,* Sentry ed. (Boston: Houghton Mifflin, 1965), 1073, 15:51–56.

2. Deepak Chopra, *Life After Death: The Burden of Proof* (New York: Harmony Books, 2006), 179.

3. Lynne Ann DeSpelder and Albert Lee Strickland, *The Last Dance: Encountering Death and Dying* (Mountain View, CA: Mayfield Publishing Company, 1999), 505.

4. Saint Paul, "Epistle to Corinthians," 15:51–56.

5. Philip Kapleau, *Zen: Down in the West* (New York: Anchor Press, 1979), 296.

6. Bill Newcott, "Life After Death," *AARP Magazine,* September–October 2007, 60.

7. Greene, *The Fabric of Cosmos,* 345.

8. Ibid., 347.

9. Gleiser, *The Prophet and the Astronomer,* 132.

10. Greene, *The Fabric of Cosmos,* 114.

11. Ibid., 90.

12. Gleiser, *The Prophet and the Astronomer,* 172.

13. Robert Naeye, "Black Hole Record Shattered," NASA Report, Goddard Space Flight Center, August 12, 2007, 2.

14. Marie-Louise von Franz, *On Death and Dreams: A Jungian Interpretation* (Boston: Shambhala, 1986), viii–ix, 156, 166–67.

15. David Hawkins, *The Eye of the I: From Which Nothing Is Hidden* (West Sedona, AZ: Veritas Publishing, 2001).

16. Campbell, *The Power of Myth,* 84, 282.

Index

ABOUT THE AUTHOR AND CONTRIBUTORS

OLGA BROM SPENCER, Ph.D., is a psychologist, author, and octogenarian practicing what she writes about: self-development. As a clinician, she was on the faculty of The New York University School of Social Work. She founded and directed the Center for Family Development, Inc. and the World Trade Family Center at the WTC, pioneering innovative treatment modalities for one-parent families, with the cooperation of Dr. William Schwarts, Margaret Mead, Marianne Walters, and Adelphi University. Her retirement led to the doctoral dissertation, *Retirement— New State of Development,* which identified factors in successful aging. Among her honors are the AARP National Award for Seniors and the Star of the Year Award for the Westport/Weston (Connecticut) AARP. *New Frontiers in Aging* is her fourth book drawing on sciences and spirituality in defining new possibilities for development in the senior years of life.

NATAN BAUMAN, Ed.D., M.S., Eng., F-AAA, is a leader in the field of hearing health care. He received a master's degree in electroacoustics and electronics from Wroclaw Polytechnic Institute in Poland and both a master's degree in Audiology and a doctoral degree in Audiology from Columbia University.

Prior to his work at his current facility, The Hearing, Balance & Speech Center, Dr. Bauman was the Director of a comparable facility at Yale–New Haven Hospital for 10 years. He also served as an Assistant Clinical

Professor at the Yale School of Medicine. In 1988, he opened The Hearing, Balance & Speech Center, and he established The New England Tinnitus and Hyperacusis Clinic in 1997. Both establishments offer patients the finest technologically advanced devices and testing procedures for their hearing health. The New England Tinnitus and Hyperacusis Clinic is the only certified treatment center in southern New England.

Dr. Bauman invented the "Totally Open Canal Hearing Aid," Vivatone. Vivatone was the first hearing aid of its kind known to eliminate hearing aid wearers' common frustrations of "feeling plugged up" or feeling as if they were in an echo chamber. Because Vivatone hearing aids allow an open ear canal, the plugged-up feeling and echo chamber are eliminated and a more natural sound is heard. Its size and ability to be worn behind the ear provides wearers with a discreet hearing aid. Because of his success with hearing aid development, Dr. Bauman opened Hearing Aid Laboratories of New England in August 2006. The Laboratory allows him to develop custom-made hearing aids for his patients.

Dr. Bauman has published numerous articles in professional journals. He is a frequent guest speaker and lecturer at audiological symposiums both nationally and internationally.

ANNA C. FREITAG, M.D., F.A.C.P., F.A.C.E., F.A.C.D.S., is a board-certified endocrinologist and Medical Director of The Stamford Hospital Diabetes & Endocrine Center, Stamford, Connecticut. She is an Assistant Clinical Professor of Medicine at the University of Connecticut School of Medicine and President of the Fairfield County (Connecticut) Leadership Council of the American Diabetes Association. She has been named one of Connecticut's Top Doctors in Endocrinology and Internal Medicine for three consecutive years by *Connecticut Magazine* and one of America's Top Physicians by the Consumers' Research Council of America for the past two years.

NANCY M. RYAN, M.S., R.D., C.D.E., is a nutrition consultant and certified diabetes educator in private practice in Greenwich, Connecticut. She received her Bachelor of Science degree, summa cum laude, in Food and Nutrition and Master of Science in Nutritional Sciences from the University of Connecticut. She has held professional positions as research dietician at the Yale–New Haven Hospital Clinical Research

Center, as well as directing clinical nutrition programs at Norwalk Hospital and the American Fitness Institute in Greenwich. As a consultant for health departments in Fairfield, Greenwich, Westport-Weston, and Stratford, she has designed and conducted community health education programs on such topics as diabetes self-management, weight loss, smoking cessation, and heart health. During her career, she has been involved with various professional and health associations including past president of the Connecticut Dietetic Association, board member of the American Heart Association Southwestern Fairfield County Branch, and member of the American Diabetes Association Leadership Council for Fairfield County.

JOEL B. SINGER, M.D., F.A.C.S., is a former New Yorker who has maintained a cosmetic surgery practice in Connecticut for the past 30 years. Dr. Singer graduated from the Yale University School of Medicine and completed his surgery and plastic surgery residence at Yale–New Haven Hospital and Rhode Island–Brown University Hospitals, respectively. He is certified by the American Board of Plastic Surgery, the American Society of Plastic Surgeons (ASPS), and the Connecticut Society of Plastic and Reconstructive Surgeons (CSPRS).

Dr. Singer provides aesthetic cosmetic services to hundreds of people every year. The practice offers natural-looking, long-lasting results, known for quality work. Dr. Singer has been at the forefront in developing the procedure known as the "weekend facelift" and other minimally invasive procedures.